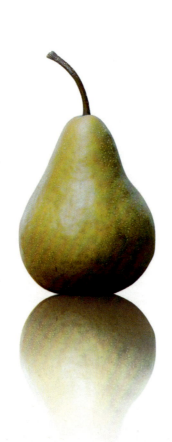

FRUIT BELLY

ROMY DOLLÉ

© 2015 Romy Dollé. All rights reserved.

Except as permitted under the United States Copyright Act of 1976, reproduction or utilization of this work in any form or by any electronic, mechanical, or other means, now known or hereafter invented, including xerography, photocopying, and recording, and in any information storage and retrieval system, is forbidden without written permission of the publisher.

Mention of specific companies, organizations, or authorities in this book does not imply endorsement by the author or publisher. Information in this book was accurate at the time researched. The author received no incentives or compensation to promote the item recommendations in the book.

Library of Congress Control Number: 2015945802
Library of Congress Cataloging-in-Publication Data is on file with the publisher
Dollé, Romy 1970 -
Fruit Belly/Romy Dollé

ISBN: 978-1-939563-21-7
1. Health 2. Weight Loss 3. Diet 4. Physical Fitness

Cover Design: Hauptmann & Kompanie Werbeagentur, Zürich
German Version Interior Design & Layout: Lars Hohmann, Dortmund
Photography: Arman Öztürk © Dave Dollé Pure Training GmbH
Additional Photography and Illustration credits: see page 229
English Version Interior Layout: Caroline De Vita
English Text Translation: Sarah Cadalbert
English Version Editor: Dolores Lusitana

Publisher: Primal Blueprint Publishing.
23805 Stuart Ranch Rd. Suite 145 Malibu, CA 90265
For information on quantity discounts, please call 888-774-6259,
email: info@primalblueprint.com, or visit PrimalBlueprintPublishing.com.

DISCLAIMER
The ideas, concepts, and opinions expressed in this book are intended to be used for educational purposes only. This book is sold with the understanding that the author and publisher are not rendering medical advice of any kind, nor is this book intended to replace medical advice, nor to diagnose, prescribe, or treat any disease, condition, illness, or injury. It is imperative that before beginning any diet program, including any aspect of the diet methodologies mentioned in *Fruit Belly*, you receive full medical clearance from a licensed physician. The author and publisher claim no responsibility to any person or entity for any liability, loss, or damage caused or alleged to be caused directly or indirectly as a result of the use, application, or interpretation of the material in this book. If you object to this disclaimer, you may return the book to publisher for a full refund.

CONTENTS

FOREWORD..8

CHAPTER 1 | QUICK FIX............................13
Quick Fix: Will It Work or Not? How To Start?..........13
When To Start The 4-Day Quick Fix......................15
Preparing and Beginning The 4-Day Quick Fix............16
Meal Plan Information..................................19
Food/Feelings Diary....................................20
What To Do After The 4-Day Quick Fix...................21
How To Interpret The Results...........................21
Decision Diagram.......................................22
Fabian and His Belly...................................23
Isabelle: Before and After The 4-Day Quick Fix.........26
Roland: Before and After The 4-Day Quick Fix...........27
"C" (age 40): Before and After The 4-Day Quick Fix.....28

CHAPTER 2 | FAT BELLY............................30
Definition Of A Bloated Belly..........................30
The Reasons For Bloating...............................31
Definition Of A Fat Belly..............................32
Dr. Torsten Albers – Visceral Fat......................32
The Reasons For Having A Fat Belly.....................34
Skinny-Fat...35
Combination Of A Bloated and Fat Belly.................35
Fecal Abdomen Shapes...................................36
Genetic Characteristics................................37

CHAPTER 3 | REASONS FOR HAVING A FAT BELLY.....40
Food Intolerances......................................40
Gluten...41
Dr. Albers – Leaky Gut Syndrome........................43
Food Intolerances: FODMAP..............................44
Are Artificial Sugars An Alternative?..................45
Natural, Calorie-Free and Calorie-Reduced Sugar........46
The Truth About Fructose (Fruit Sugar).................48
Dr. Albers – The Science Of Fructose...................50
Dr. Albers – Effects Of Consuming Too Much Fructose....53
Dr. Albers – How Is Fructose Intolerance Detected?.....55
Lactose (Milk Sugar)...................................57
What Is Lactose Intolerance?...........................58
Symptoms Of Lactose Intolerance........................59
Dr. Albers – Not Enough Calcium Without Dairy Products?....61
Histamine Intolerance..................................61
Indigestion With Raw Food..............................64
Stress...72
Exercise...76
Rest and Relaxation....................................78

CHAPTER 4 | SOLUTIONS............................80
Eliminating Bloating – Quick Fix.......................80
Lose Weight – Change Your Lifestyle....................81
Losing Body Fat – Setting Realistic Goals..............84
Body Mass Index (BMI)..................................86
Dr. Albers – How Much Body Fat Is Healthy?.............87

Strategically Change Your Lifestyle..89
Pure Food Paleo Principles..92
Drinks...96
Testimonial..98
Lose Body Fat – Implement Your Plan...................................104
Optimal Body (Belly) Posture...106
Fitness Routine: HIIT – High Intensity Interval Training...109
Dr. Albers – Strength Training And Weight Loss................111
Prioritize Relaxation..112
Dr. Albers – Lack Of Sleep And Obesity...............................115
Reduce Stress..116
Emotions...119

CHAPTER 5 | PLANNING MEALS..............................122
Meal Plan 1: Pure Food Paleo Low Carb...............................123
Meal Plan 2: Pure Food Paleo...123

CHAPTER 6 | RECIPES...126
Recipe Information..126
Breakfast..131
Apple and Coconut Muffins..132
Blueberry Coconut Muffins...132
Frittata..133
Breakfast Wrap..134
Coconut Berry Crunch Muesli..136
Beet/Carrot Smoothie..137
Carrot/Coconut Milk Smoothie..139
Beet/Avocado Smoothie..139

Breakfast Burger..140
Butter Coffee (hot)..142
Butter Coffee (cold)..143
Main Dishes...145
Zoodles with Shrimp...146
Sashimi Puzzle..148
Cold Avocado Cucumber Soup..149
Mushroom Kebabs On Potato and Celeriac Purée............150
Thai Soup...152
Tuna Salad with Vegetables..153
Spinach Topped with Salmon...154
Chicken Breast with Sweet Potato and Carrot Salad........156
Ground Beef and Tomato Stew..157
Cauliflower Steak with Poached Egg and Sweet Potato Fries...158
Paleo Burger...160
Sweet Potato Noodles with Chicken Liver..........................162
Pumpkin Soup with Chicken Breast......................................163
Fish "Packages" with Beet Salad..164
Paleo Bibimbap..166
Small Pure Food Paleo Desserts..168
Chocolate Mousse...170
Apple Topped with Crumble...171
Banana Crunch...172
Paleo Bounties...173
Macadamia Nut Cookies..174
Coffee Ice Cream...176
Berry Soup..177
Snacks..178

CHAPTER 7 | TRAINING 180
Workout Information 180
Why Is Physical Health So Important? 182
Warm-Up (A, B, C and D) 183
Loosening Muscles and Connective Tissue (E, F, G and H) 185
Stretching (I, J, K, L, M and N) 187
10-Minute High Intensity Interval Training (HIIT) - Men 190
10-Minute High Intensity Interval Training (HIIT) - Women ... 194
20-Minute High Intensity Interval Training
    (HIIT) – Men & Women 198

CHAPTER 8 | SOURCES AND INFORMATION 204
Pure Food Products 205
Pure Food Basic Information 206
Protein Powder 209
Fructose and FODMAP Food List 210
Sugar Levels 210

Appendix 214
Quick Fix Shopping List 215
Equipment Suppliers 215

Acknowledgments 216
Epilogue 220
Contributors 223
Credits 228

FOREWORD

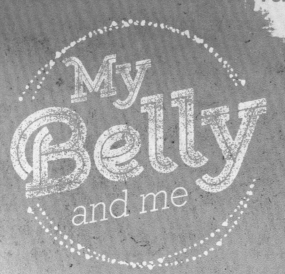

My belly and I have a long history—we go way back. I was just barely 20 years old when my troubles began. I was not happy with how my belly looked. I was thin, but I still had a belly! I followed strict diets and lost weight, but my belly just held its ground and would not go away. Every time I'd look in the mirror, there was my belly, grinning at me. I hated my belly. But my belly didn't seem to understand why I felt this way. I would say we had a love/hate relationship, my belly and me. I knew that I made a lot of decisions based on my "gut feeling," sometimes more often than using my head. Not only did I have feelings in my belly, I knew that one day it would hold my baby.

But all that I longed for was a flatter, more toned, and nicely shaped belly. Eventually I asked myself: why won't my belly work with me, instead of always against me? We had to figure out a way to work together. I read books on health, I devoured fitness magazines, and I went to doctor after doctor searching for help. I looked for the answer for years and tried everything under the sun. I got advice from specialists, I tried various tips and tricks, I drank special powered drinks and detoxing teas, I took pills, I had colon-hydrotherapy, I gave myself belly massages. Even by doing 100 crunches a day and other special exercises for years,—focusing on abs, legs, and glutes—my belly held on. I was absolutely desperate. But I was not about to give up and let my stubborn belly win. I am way too ambitious and persistent to let that happen.

Today, 25 years later, I love my belly. I am so proud of my belly and of myself. After so many years, we have finally found each other. No, it wasn't my pregnancy that made this possible. While I was pregnant, I gave my belly a break, but only until the day of the birth and not a moment longer. Experimentation showed me the way that my body would like to be nourished so that everything could function smoothly. Over the past ten years, I was able to put the puzzle together piece by piece to find my physical and mental wellbeing.

YOUR BELLY AND YOU

With this book, I'd like to help you find your way to feeling better faster and more efficiently. You don't necessarily need a six-pack in order to be happy; maybe you'd just like to give your belly a rest and have regular, problem-free bowel movements. Whatever your goal is, this book will help you become friends with your belly.

In the process of working on your belly, maybe you think it's unnecessary to avoid eating foods containing gluten, such as bread, pasta, and beer. These foods are not only delicious, but are also quite inexpensive. They seem to make life easier when you're in the company of friends or family, at parties, or in restaurants, where you may feel uncomfortable with your special dietary needs or wishes.

Maybe you have decided, despite your balloon belly, to not give up eating large amounts of fruits, salads, and/or dairy products. This is your decision. But you should really be kind to your belly and give your belly some credit. You belly has been made into an involuntary garbage can and suffers from horrible bloating, pressure, and pain. Your belly has taken the job of working overtime on tasks that it simply cannot continue doing without unpleasant symptoms. Be kind and loving to your belly as long as it is working as well as it can. Not every belly has the strength to digest large amounts of raw food. You are most likely receiving clear

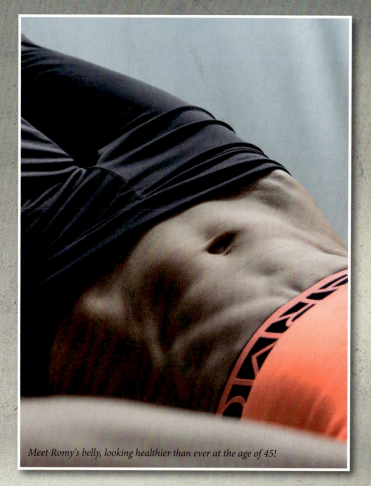

Meet Romy's belly, looking healthier than ever at the age of 45!

FOREWORD

signals that your belly is overwhelmed with too much salad, raw vegetables, and fruit. You are ignoring what your body is trying to tell you when you should be treating yourself with respect.

Continuing this way will not make you happy and content. Either you change your diet and figure out what your body can easily digest and tolerate, or you accept your balloon belly and surrender to feeling uncomfortable. Making changes may seem too tedious and time-consuming, but it's worth it in the end. As the old saying goes: "A pig will eat everything." This is true about the domestic pig up to a certain point. The poor pig doesn't really have a choice in what he eats. He eats what he is given. We, on the other hand, are in charge of our own decisions. We eat what we want, with full knowledge: food containing artificial additives, way too much sugar, fast food, energy drinks, and products containing gluten. We smoke, we drink alcohol, we don't get enough sleep, we are stressed out, and we are sick. We go to the doctor and get medicine to treat the symptoms. We complain and whine and moan. We are completely stressed and unsatisfied. We are in bad moods and everyone around us is affected by our unhappiness. It's our choice, our decision. We set the priorities in our lives. We are not able to change everything, but we are able to change a lot.

My advice to you is intended as a foundation, so that you won't have to spend years on end like I did to finally get rid of your

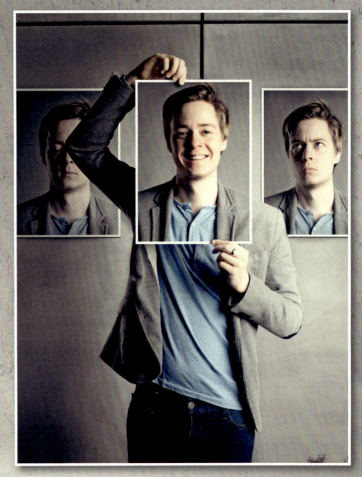

FRUIT BELLY

"unloved" belly. You can improve your digestion and get your body in better shape. I will give you practical tips for your everyday life on how to optimize your diet step by step. I will explain to you what—besides your diet—has an influence on your weight, your digestion, and the shape your body is in, and how everything is connected in the end. Depending on your starting point and your health, you may experience immediate results. Please don't be disappointed, though, if it takes a bit longer to see any positive changes. You'll need quite a lot of discipline and some patience. In theory, it's easy to change your habits. In reality, however, it's a bit more complicated to make a change, and it will take at least 60 days until a new habit becomes automated.

Once you understand the connection and recognize what is happening in your body, my advice for this new lifestyle will all make sense. It will be easier for you to follow and you'll feel better and lighter. You will experience many "aha!" moments when you eat consciously and observe how your body reacts to the food it's been given. Some of these moments may be when you don't feel well, have a foggy head, and/or get headaches when you eat something containing gluten. It may also be that you experience relief when your stomach muscles are finally visible because you have been eating fewer raw foods. One of my biggest "aha!" moments was when my bloating went away and my stomach was actually flat just a few days after I stopped eating fruit. I didn't know if I should laugh or cry. I finally knew the cause of my problems. I read up on sugar and fructose. I now know that sugar and fructose are like drugs. They produce patterns in your brain similar to marijuana, heroin, alcohol, and nicotine. Sugar and fructose also inhibit your body from losing fat. They raise your blood sugar and cause cravings. They make you fat, moody, and unsatisfied. The result is metabolic syndrome and its four characteristic factors: abdominal obesity, high blood pressure, abnormal blood lipids, and insulin resistance.

Do I want to be addicted? Do I want to have digestive problems and be bloated all the time? Do I want to endanger myself with metabolic syndrome? The answer was, and is, very simple: no.

For almost five years now, I no longer eat fruit, with the exception of avocado and sometimes a small portion of berries. Do I miss fruit? No. Do I miss the vitamins and fiber found in fruit? No. I eat a variety of vegetables and have a choice of eating a huge selection of healthy, natural fats and protein (animal and vegetarian). I place great emphasis on seasonal, local, and organic food. I get animal products, when possible, from animals that were humanely reared and fed. My blood levels are better than they've ever been. I haven't been sick in the past five years. I have a lot more energy. I sleep well and I feel well-balanced. My life is fun, even on days when not everything goes as smoothly as it should.

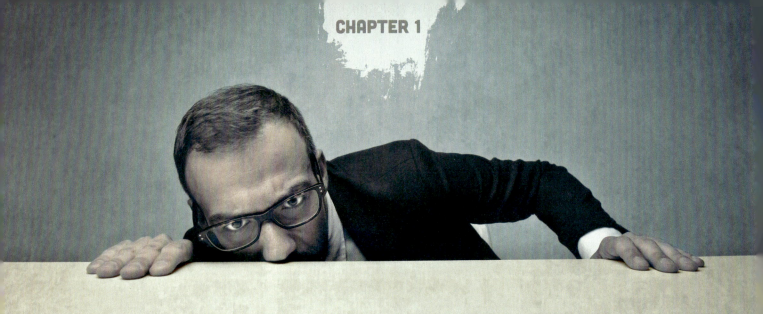

QUICK FIX: WILL IT WORK OR NOT? HOW TO START?

Do you want to make a change? Do you want to eliminate any digestive or other problems you may have? Do you want a nice belly? Yes? Then I have an important question for you:

Do you eat or drink these foods at least once daily?
(Check all items that apply)

If you checked more than five items in one of both charts, you can give the following 4-Day Quick Fix a try to find out if your symptoms could be the result of your eating habits.

If you checked less than five items in one or both charts, trying the Quick Fix might also be an option to see if eliminating problematic foods from your diet could lead to an improvement.

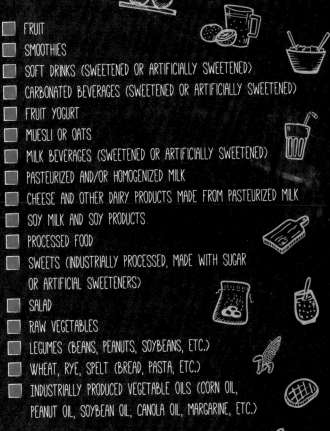

- [ ] FRUIT
- [ ] SMOOTHIES
- [ ] SOFT DRINKS (SWEETENED OR ARTIFICIALLY SWEETENED)
- [ ] CARBONATED BEVERAGES (SWEETENED OR ARTIFICIALLY SWEETENED)
- [ ] FRUIT YOGURT
- [ ] MUESLI OR OATS
- [ ] MILK BEVERAGES (SWEETENED OR ARTIFICIALLY SWEETENED)
- [ ] PASTEURIZED AND/OR HOMOGENIZED MILK
- [ ] CHEESE AND OTHER DAIRY PRODUCTS MADE FROM PASTEURIZED MILK
- [ ] SOY MILK AND SOY PRODUCTS
- [ ] PROCESSED FOOD
- [ ] SWEETS (INDUSTRIALLY PROCESSED, MADE WITH SUGAR OR ARTIFICIAL SWEETENERS)
- [ ] SALAD
- [ ] RAW VEGETABLES
- [ ] LEGUMES (BEANS, PEANUTS, SOYBEANS, ETC.)
- [ ] WHEAT, RYE, SPELT (BREAD, PASTA, ETC.)
- [ ] INDUSTRIALLY PRODUCED VEGETABLE OILS (CORN OIL, PEANUT OIL, SOYBEAN OIL, CANOLA OIL, MARGARINE, ETC.)

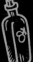

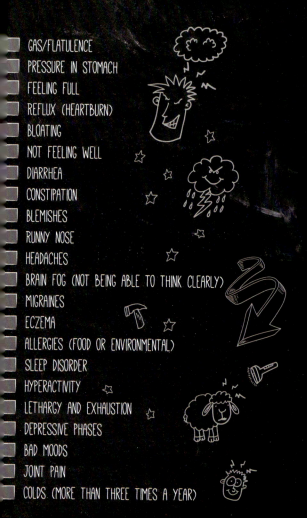

- GAS/FLATULENCE
- PRESSURE IN STOMACH
- FEELING FULL
- REFLUX (HEARTBURN)
- BLOATING
- NOT FEELING WELL
- DIARRHEA
- CONSTIPATION
- BLEMISHES
- RUNNY NOSE
- HEADACHES
- BRAIN FOG (NOT BEING ABLE TO THINK CLEARLY)
- MIGRAINES
- ECZEMA
- ALLERGIES (FOOD OR ENVIRONMENTAL)
- SLEEP DISORDER
- HYPERACTIVITY
- LETHARGY AND EXHAUSTION
- DEPRESSIVE PHASES
- BAD MOODS
- JOINT PAIN
- COLDS (MORE THAN THREE TIMES A YEAR)

You will not lose body fat with the 4-Day Quick Fix. If you'd like to safely and sustainably lose body fat, please refer to Chapter 4 and the chapters following.

The Quick Fix is designed to reduce and excrete excess water retention and bloating (gas in the digestive tract). The Quick Fix diet days will soothe digestion and allow the digestive organs (stomach, intestines, liver, and kidneys) to recover and rejuvenate.

During these four days, you are to completely avoid eating any raw foods (including fruits) as well as milk and other dairy products, grains, soy, legumes, eggs, artificial sweeteners, and industrial plant oils. These foods are the main cause of digestive disorders and food intolerances. By eliminating these foods from your diet, you'll most likely see great improvements in your symptoms. This really is possible by doing the Quick Fix for just four days.

As you can see in the diagrams of our people being tested, you are able to lose weight (from less fluid retention/edema) and reduce your waist measurements (from less bloating/gas in the intestines). You'll feel much lighter, you'll have much more energy, and you'll sleep better. Your body will enjoy the break without going hungry. Your digestion will be able to do its job

FRUIT BELLY

more easily. Everything that you eat in these four days is, for most people, easily digestible and filling (satiating), and provides all the necessary nutrients.

Try it and you can feel it yourself!

WHEN TO START THE 4-DAY QUICK FIX?

It's better if you read all the instructions thoroughly today (next section), buy all the necessary food, and begin tomorrow morning. The four days breeze by quickly and the lessons you'll learn by completing the Quick Fix can be very helpful. You will most likely notice the foods that you have avoided in the past four days are the probable reason for your bloated belly and discomfort. If there is a planned event coming up where you'll feel obligated to eat and would like to be a part of, then it's probably best you don't start right now. But try not to procrastinate and find excuses; this will not be of any help to you.

Procrastinating could also be a sign that you might be scared of the truth. You already know now that you have certain habits that aren't good for you. Maybe you just don't want to admit it, and this could be the reason you keep finding excuses to not start the Quick Fix.

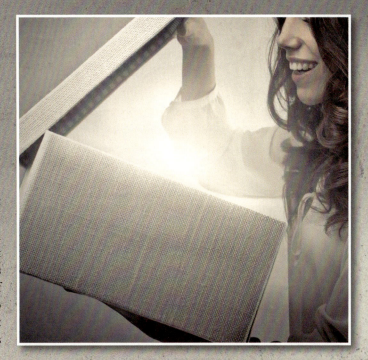

In Chapter 4, ten principles of "pure food" are described based on the Paleo diet. Read it through and then begin step by step at your own pace. It's not necessary to begin drastically; just start slowly. Your diet probably isn't the only cause of your symptoms. A healthy lifestyle must include the following points: diet, exercise, relaxation/free-time, and social environment. You'll find a

CHAPTER 1 | QUICK FIX

lot of information on this in Chapter 3, and you'll find the ways to solve any of these problems in Chapter 4.

You can begin to optimize your lifestyle anytime, anywhere.

> **EVEN THE LONGEST JOURNEY BEGINS WITH ONE SMALL STEP.**
> — Chinese proverb

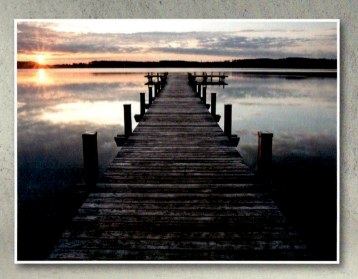

PREPARING AND BEGINNING THE 4-DAY QUICK FIX

- **Read all the information on pages 13 to 22**

- **Buy all the necessary food** (you'll find a shopping list at the end of the book in the appendix)

- **Weigh and measure yourself:**
  - Weigh yourself first thing in the morning after going to the bathroom, before eating breakfast or drinking anything (preferably naked or in your underwear)
  - Measure the circumference of the largest part of your waist using a flexible tape measure (just try to remember where exactly you measured—you could also take a picture of where you measured)
  - Take a picture of your belly

- **Begin with the eating plan**

- **Keep a food/feelings diary**

- **Always eat dinner before 8:00 pm**

FRUIT BELLY

- **Stick to an evening ritual**
  - Take a warm bath with Epsom salt, or have a warm footbath followed by massaging your feet with magnesium oil or cream.
  - Drink a cup of chamomile tea or herbal evening tea, read a relaxing book, take an evening stroll, watch a soothing movie, do some stretching, or use a massage roller to treat yourself to a massage.
  - Go to bed by 10:00 pm. Your bedroom should be completely dark: no lights or lamps, TV, or electrical devices, and your iPhone should be on airplane mode; temperature should not exceed 65° F.
  - In most cases, falling asleep will not be difficult. You may find the first night a bit challenging if you slept in later that morning.
  - When you get up in the morning, either by your alarm going off or waking up on your own, open your windows and let in the morning light and fresh air. Turn your body on to "awake mode."

- **Fitness training/exercise**
  - Fitness training is optional
  - Exercise is mandatory—a 30 to 60 minute walk outside in the fresh air daily

- Repeat the above for days two through four

- **On the fifth day, measure and weigh yourself again (see instructions in the third point on this list)**

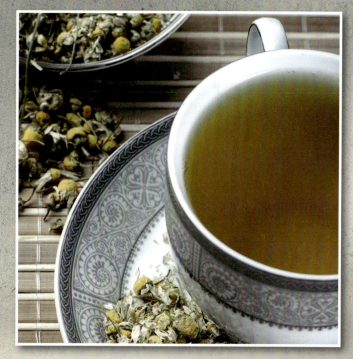

4-DAY QUICK FIX MEAL PLAN

	BREAKFAST	LUNCH	DINNER	SNACK (OPTIONAL)
DAY 1	Beet/Carrot Smoothie	Chicken Breast with Sweet Potato Carrot Salad	Spinach Topped with Salmon	½ portion of breakfast, lunch, or dinner
DAY 2	8:00 am Butter Coffee 10:00 am Butter Coffee	Ground Beef and Tomato Stew	Mushroom Kebabs on Celeriac/Potato Puree	½ portion of breakfast, lunch, or dinner
DAY 3	Carrot/Coconut Milk Smoothie	Thai Soup	Sweet Potato Noodles with Chicken Liver	½ portion of breakfast, lunch, or dinner
DAY 4	Beet/Avocado Smoothie	Tuna Salad with Vegetables	Pumpkin Soup with Chicken Breast	½ portion of breakfast, lunch, or dinner

All Meal Plan recipes in this book can be found on pages 132-178

MEAL PLAN INFORMATION

- Each meal can be substituted (breakfast, lunch, or dinner) with the exception of the butter coffee.
- Drink butter coffee (see pages 142-143) only at breakfast. Butter coffee can also replace a snack (but only before noon).
- You may drink an espresso without milk and sugar (and without alternative sweeteners).
- Don't drink any coffee after 2:00 pm.
- Allowed drinks include: water (non-carbonated) and black or herbal tea without sugar or alternative sweeteners.
- All other drinks during these four days are not allowed.
- If you're hungry between meals, you may have a half portion of one of the meals as a snack (with the exception of butter coffee, only in the mornings).
- It's wise to cook more than one portion of a meal at a time and keep it in the refrigerator.
- You may also eat the same meals every day or eat the same meal for lunch and dinner if you wish to do so.
- If you are very hungry, it is also possible to eat one-and-a-half portions of the meal.
- Don't just eat a part of the meal; eat the meal as a whole. And it's important not to leave out the meat/fish (protein).
- Don't add any other ingredients to the meals (like, onions or garlic).
- You may use salt, pepper, and herbs (fresh or dried) if desired.

Vegetarian options:

- Replace instant gelatin powder with vegetarian protein powder (reference source in the appendix).
- Replace meals with shakes (breakfast, lunch, or dinner) during the 4-Day Quick Fix.
- Eggs are not an alternative to meat, fish, or poultry because a lot of people have an intolerance to them (especially conventional varieties) and respond with inflammation or bloating.
- Soy, tofu, and legumes are also not protein alternatives. Legumes are difficult to digest and promote the formation of gas and bloating. Soy and tofu affect our hormones (especially the production of estrogen).
- Leaving out the protein part of the meal is also not an option, because the meals are designed specifically to keep you satiated.

FOOD/FEELINGS DIARY

Keeping a food/feelings diary will help you get to know yourself better and take a closer look at your eating habits. It may also help you see habits you may not even know about. By writing down your feelings, you'll be able to find out what triggers these habits.

DATE	TIME	PLACE	HUNGER	HOW YOU FEEL BEFORE YOU ATE	WHAT YOU ATE	SATIETY LEVEL	HOW YOU FEEL AFTER YOU ATE	SYMPTOMS
06/30 *(EXAMPLE)*	7:00 AM	AT HOME AT THE KITCHEN TABLE	3	STILL TIRED, NERVOUS ABOUT THE MEETING	CARROT/COCONUT MILK SMOOTHIE	7	RESTLESS, IRRITATED, ATE TOO QUICKLY	BLOATED, DIARRHEA

Hunger and satiety scale

0: Fasting "numbness", not feeling hungry anymore
1: Very hungry with food cravings
2: Headache, irritable, shaky, tired, and dizzy
3: Stomach is empty, growling occasionally; I should eat soon
4: Not feeling satisfied; food still looks good and tempting
5: Feeling content; I could eat more but I could also let it be
6: Pleasantly full; still feel satisfied after 30 minutes
7: Uncomfortably full; I ate too much
8: Bloated, noticeable protruding stomach
9: Nauseous, accompanied by stomach and backache
10: Very full; close to vomiting

The goal is to be within the 3 to 6 range

WHAT TO DO AFTER THE 4-DAY QUICK FIX

The results on day five were::

SURPRISINGLY POSITIVE

- lost 2 to 7 lbs
- 2 to 4 inches less waist circumference
- more energy and feel great

POSITIVE

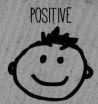

- lost approx. 2 lbs
- 0.5 to 1 inch less waist circumference
- full of energy and feel better

UNCHANGED

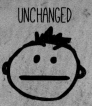

- no weight lost
- waist circumference remained the same
- tired and no motivation

HOW TO INTERPRET THE RESULTS

If you lost a significant amount of weight during these four days, it was most likely from water. This could be because of the reduced amount of carbohydrates you ate and/or the reduction of your stress level (you may have slept more and better and been more relaxed). It could also be that you have omitted the foods you have an intolerance to and that trigger water retention in your body. Reduced waist circumference is probably because you didn't eat any gas-forming foods in the past four days.

What you see now is reality. If you're nice and slim, then your belly is most likely gone or at least a lot smaller.

If you're overweight, then you now know how much of your belly is body fat. To get rid of this, you will need a lot longer than the 4-Day Quick Fix. It is necessary to make long-term diet changes and you will have to change your lifestyle. You can find more detailed information in the following chapters.

If you feel a positive change after the four days but perhaps didn't lose much weight or notice any visible changes in the circumference of your waist, I'm sure you at least feel a positive change in your digestion and your well-being. Maybe you don't have any more headaches, or stomachaches, or joint pain. And maybe you have more energy and sleep better.

Depending on your starting point and your ailments, it could be that your body just needs a bit more time to cleanse and recover. But just remember, you are on the right track.

Maybe it's not necessarily your diet that's the main problem, but other factors such as stress, a chronic lack of sleep, or an illness. We'll go deeper into this in the following chapters.

If you didn't notice any changes or improvements at all after the 4-Day Quick Fix, you will most likely feel quite frustrated, especially if you strictly followed the plan. It's completely all right to add on a few more days to the Quick Fix to see if you may just need a bit more time to notice a difference.

If you still don't notice a difference, I would recommend going to a specialist for an evaluation.

> IT COULD ALSO BE THAT YOU HAVE AN INTOLERANCE TO ONE OR MORE OF THE FOODS IN THE 4-DAY QUICK FIX. PLEASE REFER TO CHAPTER 3 UNDER FODMAPS.

DECISION DIAGRAM

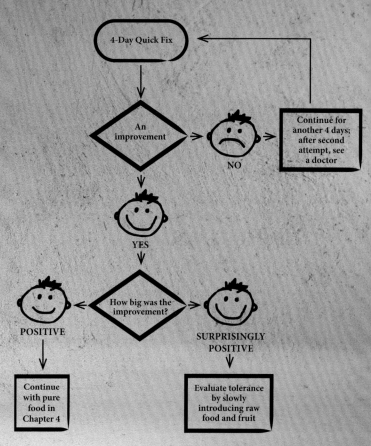

FABIAN AND HIS BELLY

Fabian is a personal trainer and is very conscious of his body. He watches what he eats and works out on a regular basis. Sometimes when his clients tell him that they would like to lose body fat, he simply can't empathize with them. He doesn't understand how difficult it can be to lose weight. He can't relate to them, since he has never had a problem with his weight in his whole life. He can't speak from experience; he can only give them theoretical tips on how to lose weight efficiently.

After thinking about it for a long while, he decided to begin an experiment in September 2013. His experiment was to gain as much body fat as possible by the end of the year and then lose the weight he had put on. He wanted to prove to himself and to his clients that by applying his tips on fitness and nutrition, that it is indeed very feasible and realistic in everyday life to lose those unwanted pounds.

For three months, from September until the end of December, Fabian ate enormous amounts of food. The biggest change he made was increasing his carbohydrate intake. Here's an example of one of his lunches: 14 ounces of spaghetti (cooked), 7 ounces of cooked minced beef, three tomatoes, one whole ball of mozzarella, and a half liter of Coca-Cola.

The plan was to gain the weight in a controlled and healthy way, but he admits that after a short time, he completely lost control. His appetite increased disproportionally, and because of all the carbohydrates he was eating (especially sugar), he experienced hunger fits and cravings that he satisfied with binge eating.

He gained 30 pounds in three months. According to the before and after body fat analysis, he gained nearly exclusively body fat, not muscle, even though he trained regularly while he was doing this experiment.

How did Fabian feel during the time he was gaining all this weight? "My belly was so bloated. It was always in the way when I tied my shoes or tried to put my pants on. This really bothered me and I just didn't feel comfortable." He was horribly afraid of getting stretch marks. "I used pregnancy creams every day from the beginning on," Fabian says with a grin. His fat belly bothered him more than he ever imagined and made his life difficult. After a while, something else caught Fabian by surprise. Not only did the extra weight make his life more physically demanding, he also suffered mentally and emotionally. He felt more and more disturbed.

In his words: "I was a bit depressed, I didn't feel well, and I'd get annoyed about mundane things. I was mentally down. Everyone looked at me strangely. Sometimes people would make jokes while I was eating. From the beginning of the experiment, I published my "progress" on Facebook. And yet, I didn't feel

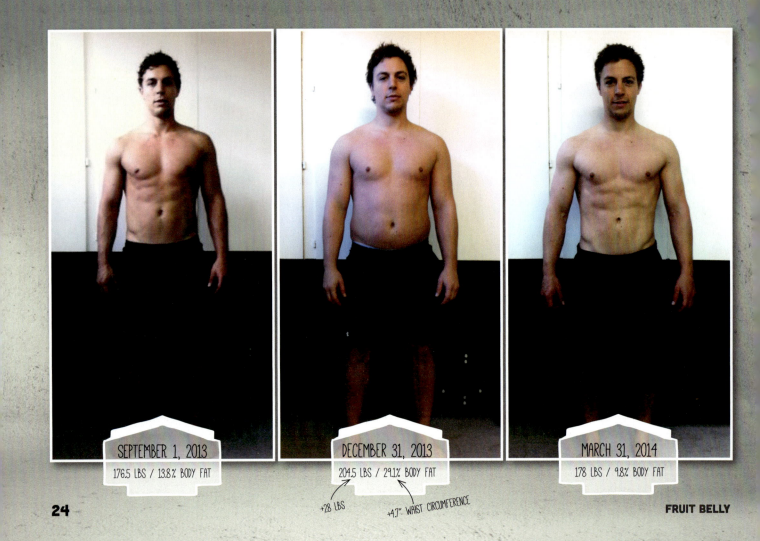

well in my own skin and for the first time in my life, I didn't feel at home in my body." When Fabian couldn't hide the weight gain any more, it was Fabian's girlfriend who would explain to the curious people that it's "just" an experiment he's doing.

JANUARY 1ST LAUNCHED THE SECOND PHASE OF THE EXPERIMENT: REMOVE THE 30 POUNDS AND RETURN TO A SIX-PACK STOMACH

As January 1, 2014 approached, Fabian could hardly wait to start the second phase of his experiment—to lose the 30 pounds he gained and to get his six-pack back. "On January 1st at 10:00 am, I went jogging and I only ate vegetables and meat for three weeks (a maximum of 1000 calories). This is how I lost the first six pounds." He was aiming for 10 pounds, though, and this only inspired him to keep going strong. With a more moderate carbohydrate diet, he was able to lose two to three pounds a week. Fabian hadn't had a sip of alcohol in three months and trained six times a week.

Fabian didn't have to do the second phase of his experiment alone. He urged his clients and his fans on Facebook to join him on his challenge to lose weight. Even though he gained most of the weight in his belly, the first place he lost weight was in his face. This goes to show, yet again, that body fat loss cannot be selectively controlled.

What was more difficult for Fabian, gaining or losing the weight? "Mentally and emotionally, gaining the weight was more difficult. I had a hard time looking at myself in the mirror. My belly bothered me, I felt depressed and in a bad mood, and I got easily annoyed. It was as if I was almost a totally different person." In contrast, losing the weight was quite easy. "I had a plan, I trained regularly, and I ate low carb food—what it took was a lot of discipline. I never felt hungry and my depressive moods disappeared after a few weeks."

After 14 weeks, Fabian is at his starting weight again. He has his beloved six-pack back.

"ACTUALLY, GAINING THE WEIGHT WAS MORE DIFFICULT," FABIAN SAYS TODAY

Conclusion: "I can empathize with overweight people much better now. I have a much better understanding of the vicious cycle you can get yourself into. With a plan and some preparation, it should be possible to lose weight—lose weight without going hungry and getting trapped in a yo-yo pattern." Fabian is convinced that he has become a better and more understanding fitness trainer by carrying out this experiment. He appreciates his body and his health a lot more now than he did before the experiment.

Would he do it again? "No, not as extreme," he says with a smile.

ISABELLE: BEFORE AND AFTER THE 4-DAY QUICK FIX

The 4-Day Quick Fix was a success with Isabelle. She lost weight and reduced her waist circumference.

Besides the motivating results, Isabelle felt great, had more energy, and finally didn't have any cravings for sweets. She will continue eating a lower-carbohydrate Paleo diet to reduce body fat.

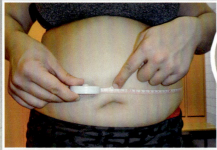

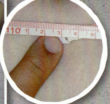

September 22, 2014
45" waist circumference / 213 lbs

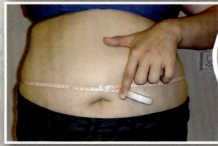

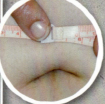

September 26, 2014
42.5" waist circumference / 206.5 lbs

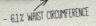

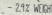

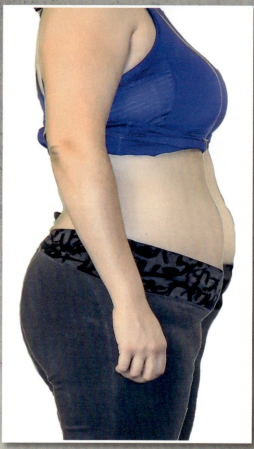

Isabelle Before and After the 4-Day Quick Fix

ROLAND: BEFORE AND AFTER THE 4-DAY QUICK FIX

Roland felt very good after the 4-Day Quick Fix. He was not completely satisfied with the only slightly improved results. He continued on, consistently doing the Quick Fix. After 20 days, he lost 7.7 lbs (3.6 percent) and had a 1.7-inch waist circumference reduction (4.1 percent).

He thought the Quick Fix meals tasted good and he felt full of energy. He wasn't hungry between meals and had no desire for sweets or alcohol.

Roland will continue on with the Paleo diet to sustainably lose body fat.

OCTOBER 2, 2014
220 LBS / BELLY 42.7"

OCTOBER 7, 2014
217.4 LBS / BELLY 42.1"

OCTOBER 23, 2014
212.3 LBS / BELLY 41"

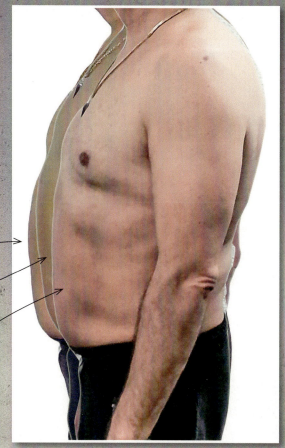

Roland Before and After the 4-Day Quick Fix

CHAPTER 1 | QUICK FIX

"C" (AGE 40): BEFORE AND AFTER THE 4-DAY QUICK FIX

She is a successful endurance runner and is very thin (13 percent body fat) except in her lower abdomen, which strongly protrudes. She eats a lot of raw food and a lot of vegetables.

After four days, the upper abdomen is even slimmer and the lower abdomen isn't as hard, but it is still distended. C. decides to continue on another four days of the diet, but there are no significant improvements. She will now go to the doctor to help find the reason for her unnatural belly shape.

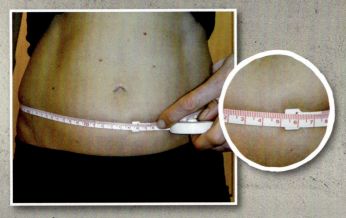

September 22, 2014
120 lbs / waist circumference 30.5"

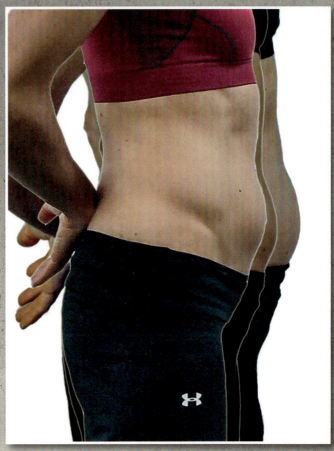

"C" (age 40): Before and After the 4-Day Quick Fix

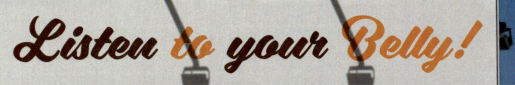

CHAPTER 2

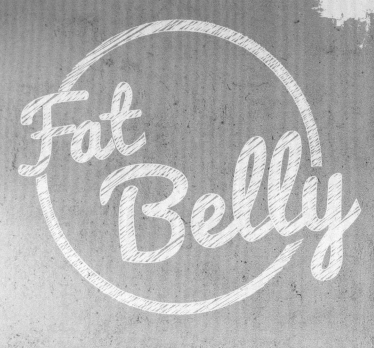

This chapter explains the differences between a bloated belly versus a fat belly, the varieties of belly shapes, and how a belly can be bloated and fat at the same time. By now, you may already know a few of these reasons. There will be more detailed information about the causes in the next chapter.

DEFINITION OF A BLOATED BELLY

A bloated belly is characterized by a swollen and protruding abdomen and is caused by the accumulation of gas in the digestive tract or stomach, or in a few cases, in the peritoneal cavity. In medical terms, bloating is also called meteorism and may be accompanied by flatulence, although gas is not necessarily released when suffering from meteorism.

Gas is produced during each process of digestion. This occurs for many different reasons. Sometimes a bit of air is swallowed while eating. The faster you eat, the more air you could accidentally swallow. Swallowing up to half a gallon a day is within the normal range.

Gas is also produced in your intestines. In this case, it's the intestinal bacteria that are the cause. It's hard to imagine the amount of intestinal bacteria we have, exceeding the number of somatic cells by ten times. As with our somatic cells, intestinal bacteria also have their own metabolism (producing methane, hydrogen, nitrogen, and carbon dioxide). Fermented gas, such as hydrogen sulfate, may also be produced in small amounts.

It is particularly important that the intestines are able to absorb the gas. Most of the time, the gases are reabsorbed into the bloodstream through the intestinal walls, and are exhaled through the lungs. This explains why your belly is flat again in the morning if you experienced bloating the night before. In this case, the intestinal gases were excreted through the lungs, which then in turn can cause you to have a bad taste in your mouth in the morning, also known as "morning breath." Whatever gas is not absorbed by the intestinal mucosa is later excreted as flatulence.

Sometimes bloating is completely harmless and will go away on its own after some time. In other cases, it could be that it does not go away so quickly and becomes chronic, causing painful symptoms. These symptoms include: irregular bowel movements, constipation, tension and a feeling of fullness, sharp pains in the upper and lower abdomen, and peristaltic sounds (gurgle-gurgle). In some cases, additional symptoms may be present, such as nausea, vomiting, and diarrhea.

Very often, a bloated belly will feel very hard to the touch and is very sensitive. Discomfort is worsened mostly when in the sitting position or when wearing tight-fitting clothes.

Many suffering from these symptoms find it difficult to take their mind off their midsection, concentrating only on the uncomfortable way they feel. This in turn affects their overall mental, physical, and spiritual wellbeing. Focusing on everyday tasks and participating in social events becomes extremely difficult.

THE REASONS FOR BLOATING

1) IMPROPER DIET
(too much raw food, fruit, dairy products, sugar and artificial sweeteners, etc.)

2) FOOD INTOLERANCE
(an intolerance to fructose, lactose, histamine, gluten, etc.)

3) SWALLOWING TOO MUCH AIR WHILE EATING AND DRINKING

4) CHEWING GUM

5) STRESS

6) LACK OF SLEEP

7) DISTURBED INTESTINAL FLORA

8) PARASITES

9) FUNGI (CANDIDA)

... ETC.

DEFINITION OF A FAT BELLY

Adipose tissue in humans has the function of protecting organs and storing energy. Excess energy from food will be stored by the body in the form of fat. In times of famine, the body is then able to turn to the reserves for energy. This made complete sense in times when there was a scarcity of food. But in an affluent society, where food is everywhere and always available ("food to go," "takeout," etc.), we tend to hang on to our fat reserves, accumulating fat bellies and a bit too much padding on the hips. All fat is not equal. Our body consists of different types of fat.

DR. TORSTEN ALBERS – VISCERAL FAT

Visceral fat (also known as intra-abdominal fat) refers to the fat in the abdominal area that is stored between the organs and is therefore not directly visible. How much visceral fat we have is individual, but averages about 50 percent dependent on the person's genetics. A typical example of this form of fat is a so-called "beer belly"—a discernible protruding belly consisting of a layer of subcutaneous fat not palpable since it is located under a layer of muscle tissue.

You can measure the circumference of the waist to find the amount of visceral adipose tissue you have. This is measured just above the lateral palpable pelvic bone while breathing normally. The higher the waist circumference, the greater amount of adipose tissue in the abdomen you'll have. Studies have proven that exceeding the limit (31 inches in women and 37 inches in men) puts you at higher risk for health problems. With a circumference over 34 inches in women and over 41 inches in men, you have a much higher risk of developing type 2 diabetes, premature heart attacks, and strokes. Statistically, the mortally rate is significantly greater in people with high waist circumferences. A good way to look at it: having a waist within the normal range is like having good life insurance.

There are quite a few differences found when comparing visceral fat to subcutaneous fat. Visceral fat is very active in the constant release of fatty acids into the bloodstream. As a result of this high metabolic activity, people with increased amounts of visceral fat have increased blood lipid levels. So-called ectopic fat deposition is mainly shown in the liver and pancreas, and is now regarded as the cause for type 2 diabetes. Thus, increased abdominal fat is regarded as a sign of unfavorable fat accumulation in internal organs, which is problematic and could cause complications and illnesses.

In addition, visceral fat is very hormonally active, much more than the "sluggish" subcutaneous fat. Depending on its volume, it sends out many messages with adverse effects on the metabolism. In people who have a "beer belly," inflammatory substances are released into the bloodstream, sending signals that in turn negatively affect sugar and cholesterol metabolism. This forces hormone-like substances into the blood, resulting in blood clotting, thrombosis, high blood pressure, and other unfavorable metabolic changes. This is the reason that people with large waist circumferences are more vulnerable to these so-called internal diseases. Health-wise, a reduction in waist circumference within the normal range is more important than just losing weight to reach a normal body mass index (BMI). Therefore, thin people with above normal waist circumferences are at greater health risk than larger people with normal waist measurements.

The most important risk factors contributing to an increased amount of abdominal fat are, besides genetic predisposition, unfavorable eating habits, and lack of exercise/physical activity. Inactivity and excessive calories in your diet lead many people to a "comfort belly." In this case, men are more affected than women. Since men have more of the male sex hormones, such as testosterone, they tend to accumulate more fat in the abdominal region. Women have more of the sex hormone estrogen, which tends to distribute fat differently, storing more subcutaneous fat in the buttocks and thighs.

From a health point of view, the female fat distribution is more favorable because in the "problem areas," subcutaneous fat produces fewer harmful signal substances than visceral fat. During menopause, estrogen levels drop dramatically, which in turn can affect fat distribution in an unhealthy way, redistributing it towards the belly. Many women over the age of 50 report that their fat has "been moved up a floor" after beginning menopause. Conversely, men often observe a decline in testosterone after the age of 40, which can lead to an increase in visceral fat and thus raise their risk of health problems.

Regardless of gender, the stress hormone cortisol, which is produced in the adrenal cortex, is considered an important risk factor because of its tendency to increase visceral fat. Issues such as stress at work, personal problems, not sleeping well, or not getting enough sleep (less than six hours a night) can lead to a chronic state of stress. Elevated levels of cortisol will eventually cause a redistribution of adipose tissue, moving it away from the extremities and towards the middle of the body. This increases the risk of developing diabetes, hypertension, and vascular disease.

THE REASONS FOR HAVING A FAT BELLY

1) **CONSUMING MORE ENERGY (CALORIES) THAN THE BODY IS EXPENDING**
2) **STRESS**
3) **LACK OF SLEEP**
4) **POOR DIET**
   (sugar, industrially produced oils, processed food, artificial additives, soft drinks, energy drinks, artificial sugar, etc.)
5) **NOT ENOUGH EXERCISE**
   ... ETC.

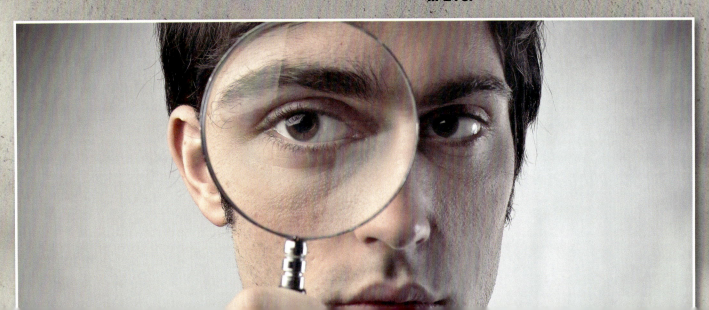

SKINNY-FAT

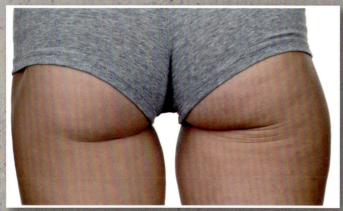

"Skinny-fat" describes people who appear to be thin with clothes on, but really have relatively high levels of body fat and very little muscle mass. They often have a little potbelly and flabby inner thighs. Skinny-fat applies to many women who eat unhealthily, tend to choose low-fat or no-fat products, and practically starve themselves to get their dream figure.

Many of these women do excessive endurance activities with the hope of looking like their idols (actresses and models in Hollywood). Unfortunately, they don't seem to realize that doing excessive endurance activities will in the long run only work against them. More muscle mass will be burned than fat, which only brings them further away from their goal.

COMBINATION OF A BLOATED AND FAT BELLY

Abdominal fat (visceral fat) and subcutaneous fat (fat that lays directly on top of muscles) will make your belly appear to be much bigger. The subcutaneous fat will cause an unattractive potbelly and hide the abdominal muscles, while visceral fat will make the whole abdominal region appear bigger. Of course, bloating amplifies it all to an even greater extent.

Normally, your organs will be standard size. There are exceptions in some cases, such as when an illness is involved. The liver, thyroid, uterus, and sometimes even the heart can become enlarged due to an illness, and sometimes even the shape of the gastrointestinal tract will change. Disorders of the gastrointestinal tract are characterized by restriction (cramps) and expansion (relaxation). When this affects larger regions of the digestive tract, the shape of the stomach may change. Chronic digestive problems can cause the shape of the stomach to change. Franz Xaver Mayr already discovered that the shape of your abdomen changes over the course of life, depending on the stage of intestinal damage, the composition of diet, and genetic makeup. For this reason, F.X. Mayr defined various belly types.

FECAL ABDOMEN SHAPES

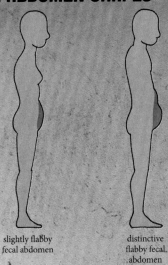
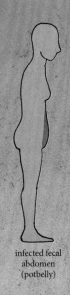
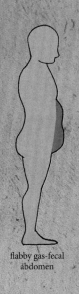
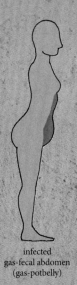

| slightly flabby fecal abdomen | distinctive flabby fecal abdomen | infected fecal abdomen (potbelly) | flabby gas-fecal abdomen | infected gas-fecal abdomen (gas-potbelly) |

For more information visit: http://www.mayr-kuren.de/mayr-kur-bauchformen.html

Note: Franz Xaver Mayr was born on November 28, 1875 in Gröbming, Austria and died on September 21, 1965 in his same city of birth. He was an Austrian gastroenterologist. He intensively dealt with the diagnosis and rehabilitation of the intestinal region, and based on his theory, developed the therapy concept F.X. Mayr cure.

Normally, a big belly is automatically associated with having a fat belly. But in reality, a pure fat belly is very rare. The size of the belly depends on how high the filling state of the intestines is. There are of course exceptions—including pregnancy, large tumors, or abnormal fluid accumulation in the abdominal cavity.

F.X. Mayr believed that accumulation of fat in the abdominal cavity is never the only cause of a protruding abdomen. F.X. Mayr also believed that there is a clear difference between a "fat belly" and "fat apron." Fat aprons are fat deposits in the abdominal wall and are relatively common. This fat often hangs down like an apron. The so-called "fat belly," however, is caused by a gas or fecal abdomen.

GENETIC CHARACTERISTICS

We are all individuals with a background of heritable genetic factors that make us unique. This is a good thing. Why do we then strive for a different body than our genetic conditions have already defined for us? If I'm 5'6" tall and have muscular legs, but I have my mind set to be 6'2" tall with the legs of a gazelle to jump higher, I'll never ever be able to accept myself and my body the way it is. As soon as you accept the fact that we all have different genetic conditions, you will then understand that we can only change our bodies to a certain extent. However, everyone is able to bring out the best in their bodies.

William Sheldon defined the constitution typology in 1942. According to these three body types, we are able to create optimal training and diet plans. In reality, most of us are not just one of the body types, but a combination of two, with one of the types being most dominant.

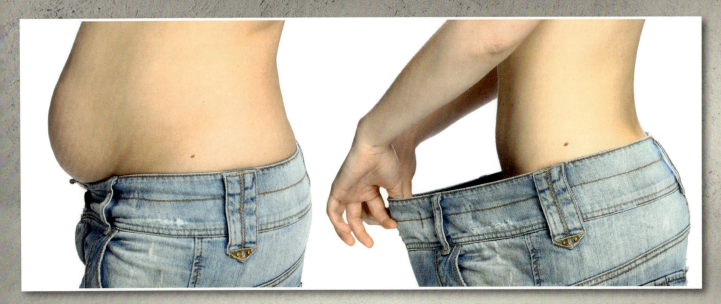

The three body types are:

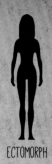
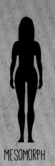

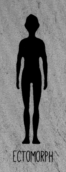
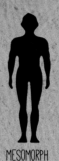
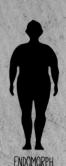

ECTOMORPH   MESOMORPH   ENDOMORPH   ECTOMORPH   MESOMORPH   ENDOMORPH

Mesomorph: muscular, athletic musculature, large chest, long torso, thick hair and skin, moderate fat reserves, able to build muscle mass easily. Mesomorphic people have their weight, for the most part, under control and only gain weight when they've eaten too much over a long period of time. They are the true "athletes" out of the three body types.

Endomorph: short arms and legs, soft musculature, wide hips, round face, thin (but a lot of) hair, dominant fat reserves, very effective muscle structure. Unfortunately, endomorphic people have a very slow metabolism and are in constant battle with obesity. These people should avoid eating a hypercaloric diet (consuming more calories than burned). Provided that there are no known intolerances, having high amounts of fat reserves in the abdominal area is common.

Ectomorph: large, long, and thin musculature, thin and less dense hair, tendency toward low fat reserves, builds up muscle very slowly ("hard gainer"). A stubborn belly is most likely due to bloating, not fat.

How Much Influence Do I Have on My Body?
No one can change their genetic body type, but with an optimal combination of training and diet, everyone has a chance at having an attractive, healthy body. Maybe not every muscle will be defined—your hips may be wider or narrower and your waist more or less pronounced—but everyone can have a nice belly, good posture, and self-confidence.

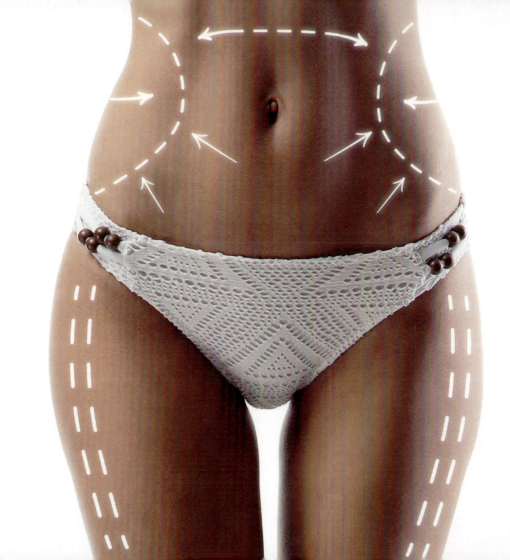

CHAPTER 3

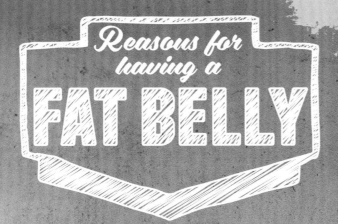
Reasons for having a FAT BELLY

Why do people have fat bellies? There are many reasons for this, but the most beautiful reason is being pregnant. Most women love their growing belly during pregnancy, Incidentally, this is the only real natural reason to have an oversized belly. Big, fat, bloated bellies are caused by malnutrition, overeating, or not eating the proper foods (or poor combination of proper food). Poor posture will also make us look fatter than we really are. Food intolerances are a common cause for making us fat and unfit. In this chapter, we'll take a look at the possible culprits behind our bloated/fat bellies.

FOOD INTOLERANCES

Here we'll talk about the most common food intolerances. In order to understand it all, we'll first give you some general information and then go into more detail about specific intolerances.

> *You have to find out for yourself how and why your gut reacts in a negative, neutral, or positive way. Each and every one of us is an individual with very unique intestinal flora (independent living organisms in our digestive tract). Only by experimenting—especially by omitting specific foods for a certain amount of time—will you be able to find out what is good and what is not so good for you.*

> *There are two different physical phenomena when dealing with food intolerances. One is when there is an allergy to foods or to certain parts of a food. The other is when there is an inability to digest a particular food or certain parts of a food.*

These two things are often confused, even though they are, in fact, completely different phenomena. With an allergy, the body's immune system plays a crucial role: the body falsely recognizes exogenous proteins as an "enemy" and produces antibodies to act as a preventative measure. Even the smallest amount of an allergy-triggering substance can cause symptoms. Celiac disease is a prime example.

With food intolerance, however, the body has lost its ability to digest a particular substance (or never actually had the ability to do so). It could be that small amounts of a certain food are tolerated because the intolerance has not yet fully developed. In some cases, only larger amounts of the substance can trigger symptoms.

GLUTEN

Gluten is a combination of different types of protein that are not only found in wheat, but also in many other grains such as spelt, rye, oats, and barley. Gluten is also found in some very ancient grains such as einkorn, khorasan, and emmer wheat (faro).

Gluten is a storage protein that provides nutrients to the seed during the process of germination. Gluten is the substance that binds the dough together so nicely when baking bread. It's adhesive. This is why it is necessary to add special binders to the dough when baking gluten-free bread, since these will replace the adhesive properties of gluten.

Gluten-free grains include millet, teff (a type of millet), and rice, as well as the so-called "pseudo grains" quinoa, amaranth, and buckwheat.

Gluten consists of two different groups, prolamines and glutelins. These differ only slightly in structure, depending on the type of grain. The typical wheat glutelin is called glutenin. The prolamine in wheat is called gliadin, in oats, avenin, and in rye secalin. Gliadin types are distinguished based on their amino acid sequences. There is not just one type of gliadin in wheat, but many different types such as the alpha, beta, gamma, and omega gliadin.

Tests for Gluten Intolerance are Often Meaningless

Testing for gluten intolerance is easier said than done. Normally, the test will look for the alpha and beta variants of gliadin antibodies, whereas gluten contains many more hazardous substances such as wheat germ agglutinin, gluteomorphin (also called gliadorphin, which is produced only by digesting gliadin), glutenin, and also the omega and gamma varieties of gliadin.

Any one or a combination of these can lead to intolerance symptoms. Thus, it is quite possible that you could be suffering from gluten sensitivity even if the gluten intolerance test results come out negative.

Gluten Sensitivity, Celiac Disease, and Gluten Intolerance—What's the Difference?

In general, "gluten sensitivity" and "gluten intolerance" are terms used to define any unfavorable reactions that may occur in connection with gluten. This would also include gluten sensitivity (celiac disease). Celiac disease (an autoimmune disease) can be easily diagnosed by means of a biopsy and certain blood markers, whereas a gluten intolerance test is not quite so simple due to the difficulties mentioned earlier.

The wide range of gluten sensitivity symptoms does not make the diagnosis any easier. While celiac disease symptoms are clear (diarrhea, stomach aches, weight loss, nutrient deficiency), gluten sensitivity will also have very similar symptoms that might not immediately indicate food intolerance. Indigestion, headaches, fatigue, sleep disorders, brain fog, problems concentrating, ADHD, ADD, autism, mood swings, dizziness, and obesity are all symptoms of gluten sensitivity, and despite all efforts are not easily relieved. Both gluten intolerances can also lead to more autoimmune diseases or possibly make existing ones even worse. This includes Hashimoto's thyroiditis (a chronically infected thyroid) and rheumatoid arthritis.

Wheat Allergies
In addition, it should be mentioned that wheat allergies often affect young children. This allergic reaction is a result of the protein in wheat, but not necessarily the proteins in other grains. Therefore, a gluten-free diet will not help all the time in this case, because wheat contains other proteins besides gluten that can also cause allergic reactions.

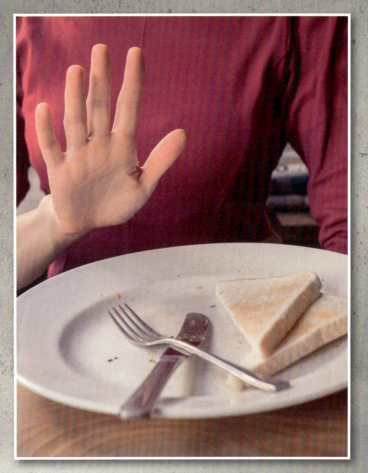

DR. TORSTEN ALBERS – LEAKY GUT SYNDROME

The intestinal mucosa barrier in humans is impermeable to the passage of completely or partially digested food particles. Through stress, excessive sports, antibiotic use, certain pain killers, alcohol, a diet high in wheat products (white bread, cereals, pasta), and a poor composition of intestinal flora, the mucosa barrier can become temporarily or permanently damaged so that partially digested food proteins and other contaminants are passed through the barrier and into the blood. This could, in turn, trigger autoimmune diseases such as rheumatic diseases or thyroid disorder. Also, allergies and other chronic inflammatory diseases in the body, such as inflammation of the liver (fatty liver disease, also known as nonalcoholic steatohepatitis), could occur.

A permanently perfect intestinal mucosa barrier is almost unheard of these days because of our lifestyles, but on the other hand, leaky gut syndrome (leaky intestinal barriers) is found more often than necessary. Unfortunately, there is currently no absolutely reliable laboratory test that can give accurate dietary reference value results by taking blood samples to diagnose a healthy gut. The determination of the protein zonulin in either serum or stool, the measuring of secretory IgA in stool, and lactulose/mannitol tests are still the best methods to diagnose leaky gut syndrome.

Therapeutically speaking, applying the use of probiotics, avoiding wheat products and alcohol, and managing stress levels are the best options for success.

Carbohydrates—Simple, Twofold, and Complex Sugars
Carbohydrates consist of sugar molecules. This does not necessarily mean that all carbohydrate-rich foods taste sweet. For example, grains (bread, pasta, rice) or potatoes do not taste sweet but they contain a lot of carbohydrates. What many people don't even consider is that fruit is very rich in carbohydrates because of the fructose content.

Depending on the number of sugar units, carbohydrates are divided into three groups:

Simple sugar (monosaccharide):
The most important representatives are dextrose (glucose) and fructose.

Twofold sugar (disaccharides):
Including primarily household sugar, malt sugar, and milk sugar. Single and twofold sugars are mainly found in candy and chocolate. They taste sweet but are empty calories that contain no vitamins or minerals and send your blood sugar levels skyrocketing.

Complex sugar (polysaccharides):
Starch is the most important polysaccharide. Complex sugar is mainly found in grains, whole-grain products, potatoes, and legumes. Blood sugar levels rise slowly after eating complex sugar.

> **Macro and Micronutrients**
> Food contains different amounts of macronutrients: carbohydrates, protein, and fat. Vitamins and minerals are micronutrients. The nutrients are broken down in the digestive tract and transported through the blood to the somatic cells to be utilized.

How Carbohydrates Function in Your Body
"Carbohydrates are broken down in the digestive tract, turning them back into simple sugar (glucose) before they enter the bloodstream," says Professor Dr. Volker Schusdziarra, head of the Clinic for Nutritional Medicine at Klinikum rechts der Isar in Munich. The hormone insulin then transports the glucose from the blood into the somatic cells. "A certain amount of glucose in the blood is essential, but it should not exceed that certain amount," explains the nutritional physician. Not enough glucose could cause hypoglycemia. Once it has dropped below a certain level, the liver must act and will begin breaking down glycogen to steady blood sugar levels. "For longer periods of hunger (starvation/famine), the liver will begin metabolizing the body's protein reserves to produce glucose. This ensures the minimal blood sugar levels in order for the brain to function properly," says Schusdziarra. This further confirms that carbohydrates are not essential for the body to function. The body is able to produce glucose out of protein through its own, a process called gluconeogenesis.

FOOD INTOLERANCES: FODMAP
Some people continue to suffer uncomfortable digestive problems despite omitting the foods they may be intolerant to. If there are no definite test results pointing at an allergy or intolerance, then you'll most likely be diagnosed with irritable bowel syndrome (IBS).

Scientists Peter Gibson and Susan Shepher at Moash University in Australia researched the reasons behind the vicious cycle of bloating, diarrhea, constipation, and discomfort. They came upon some evidence proving that certain sugars could actually be the cause of many of these ailments: "Fermentable Oligo-Di-Monosaccharides and Polyols," thus founding the term FODMAP.

Fermentable: these types of sugar have the ability and tendency to ferment in our intestines, resulting in bloating and diarrhea.
Oligosaccharides: fructans (FOS), wheat, rye, onions, garlic, galactans (GOS) (legumes), chickpeas.
Disaccharide: sucrose, maltose, and lactose.
Monosaccharide: fructose, glucose, and galactose.
Polyol: sorbitol, mannitol, xylitol, maltitol (sugar substitutes).

It is not possible to completely avoid each and every one of these types of sugar, since they are found naturally in the food we eat. It would be wise to avoid eating foods containing large amounts of these sugars for a certain amount of time, simply to see if they could be the reason behind the problems you may be experiencing.

Research has proven that there is a certain daily limit of FODMAPs that can be tolerated. If you've eaten your daily limit in lactose already, then it's no wonder that when you eat the same berries that you ate the day before with no negative effects, all of a sudden they cause you discomfort. Try picturing your FODMAP limit, applying it throughout the day, distributed evenly in each meal. If you go over your limit, then you are bound to have negative reactions.

The pure food Paleo diet eliminates the consumption of fructan and galctan by eliminating grains. Legumes are also avoided, with the occasional exception. You are able to test out fruits after a grace period, using the guide to see which fruits are better tolerated than others. It all depends on moderation. The Quick Fix not only detoxes the intestines, but also tests your individual tolerance levels.

> **Please note!** *Stress levels will also surprisingly affect FODMAP intolerance levels, since stress hormones have a heavy influence on digestion.*
>
> **Please note!** *No matter what kind of sugar we eat, our body and brain will suffer the consequences. Sugar makes us weak, unmotivated, tired, depressed, and sick.*

ARE ARTIFICIAL SUGARS AN ALTERNATIVE?

No. Need I say more? We are natural beings and we shouldn't eat anything unnatural and artificial. Our brain and body aren't so easily tricked and won't be taken for fools.

Brain scientist and diabetologist Professor Achim Peters from Lübeck, Germany also warns of the dangers of consuming artificial sweeteners. According to Peters, sweeteners discretely affect the appetite and hunger. The brain is tricked into believing that energy supplies have arrived because of the sweet taste, but artificial sweeteners do not supply any energy. So to play it safe, the brain sends out "I'm hungry" signals and turns the appetite switch on to make sure that the body gets the energy that the false energy sources promised to deliver. So even though we just ate, we get hungry again. We then supply the body with even more calories that we really don't need, and they are stored in the fat reserves. Artificial sweeteners are used in industrial farm animals to make them hungry again so they eat more, and thus get fat quicker and are able to be slaughtered earlier—adding more pounds to the scale and resulting in more profit.

Some artificial sweeteners are more harmful than others; they do not belong in the human diet and are to be avoided as much as possible.

NATURAL, CALORIE-FREE AND CALORIE-REDUCED SUGAR

Stevia

The most well known natural calorie-free sugar substitute is stevia. Stevia has been used for centuries by the indigenous people of Paraguay and Brazil in the preparation of food and beverages, and has also been used for medicinal purposes. The sweetness of dried stevia leaves is about 30 times greater than that of sugar. The advantage of using stevia is that it does not cause blood sugar levels to rise after consumption. It's important when buying stevia to check the label to make sure that there is no sugar or any other additives.

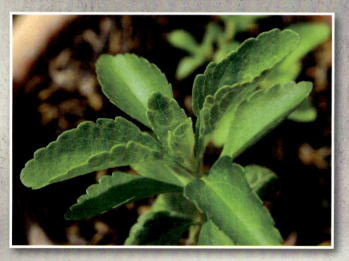

Xylitol

Xylitol (sugar alcohol) is mainly used by the food industry as a sugar substitute. It is preferred because of its known anti-cariogenic effect. Xylitol, in contrast to sugar (sucrose), is not harmful to our teeth. In fact, it has been said that it actually has a positive effect on our dental health. Xylitol has a very similar taste to normal sugar and also has the same sweetening power (for example, 1 tsp of sugar tastes like 1 tsp of xylitol). It tends to create a cooling sensation on the tongue, and when it comes in contact with saliva, it turns warm.

Similar to sorbitol, xylitol contains fewer calories than sugar. While one gram of sucrose contains 4 calories, xylitol only contains 2.4 calories per gram. Because xylitol does not require insulin to be metabolized, it is also suitable for diabetics.

Erythritol

Erythritol is also a sugar alcohol that is naturally found in pears, melons, and mushrooms. Erythritol is produced by fermentation. Yogurt, cheese, and wine are also made by using this process of fermentation. Erythritol acts as an antioxidant by binding with free radicals. The glycemic index of erythritol is zero, so it does not raise blood sugar levels. And it's calorie free.

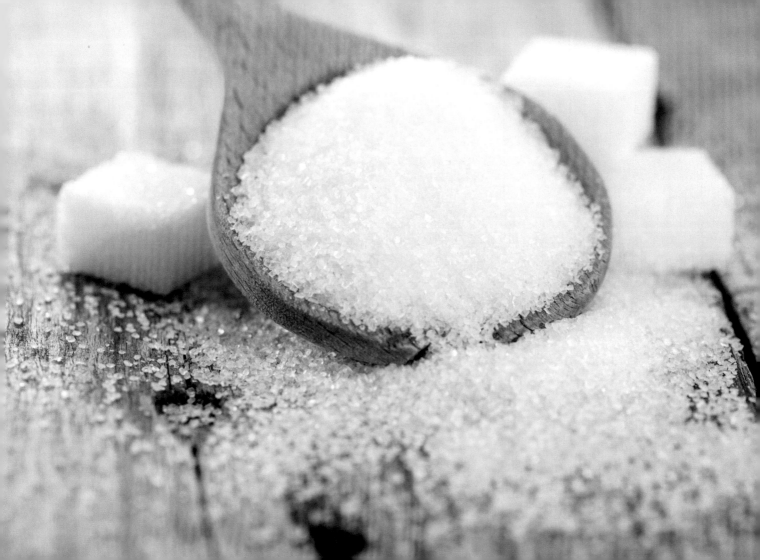

> The big disadvantage of sugar alcohols is that after consumption, they are fermented in the intestines, turned into fat molecules, and then accepted by the body as energy (fat). Because of the fermentation in the intestines, many people experience digestive problems after consuming sugar alcohols.

THE TRUTH ABOUT FRUCTOSE (FRUIT SUGAR)

In this section, we'll take a deeper look at fruit and fruit sugar. Unfortunately, fruit and its sugar are not as healthy as the advertisements from food manufacturers and the official dietary guidelines say they are.

We consume far more fruit sugar than we think we do. It's no longer just in the natural fresh fruit we eat, it's in a lot of other things, too.

- Processed food and soft drinks are sweetened with fruit sugar.
- The fructose found in processed food and drinks is no longer a natural fruit sugar as found in a banana or a pear, but much more potent. It is highly concentrated and industrially processed into what is called fruit sugar syrup or fructose syrup.
- Pure fructose is a lot sweeter than glucose (grape/corn sugar). This makes it very popular among food companies, and it's generously used in processed products and drinks.
- Fruit juice contains an overwhelming amount of fructose, since the fiber (what the whole fruit is made of) is missing. Fruit juice is just flavored sugar water.
- Dried fruits are a popular "healthy" snack and are often eaten in large amounts. What's missing here is the water that exists in fresh fruit. The concentration of fructose is considerably higher than that found in fresh fruit. Dried fruits are like candy.
- Fructose does not satiate and give you that "I'm full" feeling. Usually, shortly after eating fructose we are hungry again. (See illustration on next page.)

> HOW SUGAR STIMULATES THE APPETITE

SUGAR – THE BAD CARBOHYDRATE

Is sugar really as dangerous as alcohol or nicotine? Yes, it surely is, according to Robert Lustig, a 55-year-old professor at the University of California's Pediatric Clinic in San Francisco. He is an expert on obesity and hormone disorders in children. Through his studies and experience, the bitter truth has been revealed. Sugar is indeed a poison—a drug—similar to alcohol. It will damage the liver and cause the metabolism to become unbalanced. He has proven that it is not binging or laziness causing the rapidly increasing cases of obesity. It is, in fact, the overconsumption of sugar.

Over the past fifty years, the worldwide consumption of sugar has tripled. So have the cases of diseases of civilization, such as obesity, type 2 diabetes, and cardiovascular disorders. Nowadays, sugar is not only found in candy and sweetened beverages, it is in countless products where you would least expect it. It is in sausages, packed chicken breasts, marinated meat, bread, breakfast cereals, sauces, and the list goes on.

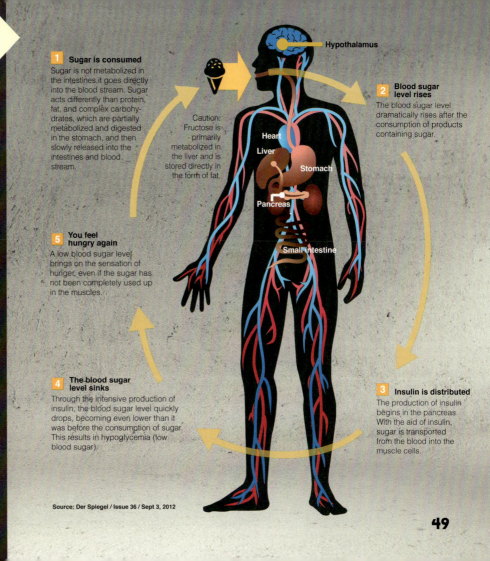

1 Sugar is consumed
Sugar is not metabolized in the intestines, it goes directly into the blood stream. Sugar acts differently than protein, fat, and complex carbohydrates, which are partially metabolized and digested in the stomach, and then slowly released into the intestines and blood stream.

Caution: Fructose is primarily metabolized in the liver and is stored directly in the form of fat.

5 You feel hungry again
A low blood sugar level brings on the sensation of hunger, even if the sugar has not been completely used up in the muscles.

4 The blood sugar level sinks
Through the intensive production of insulin, the blood sugar level quickly drops, becoming even lower than it was before the consumption of sugar. This results in hypoglycemia (low blood sugar).

2 Blood sugar level rises
The blood sugar level dramatically rises after the consumption of products containing sugar.

3 Insulin is distributed
The production of insulin begins in the pancreas. With the aid of insulin, sugar is transported from the blood into the muscle cells.

Source: Der Spiegel / Issue 36 / Sept 3, 2012

DR. ALBERS – THE SCIENCE OF FRUCTOSE

Fructose has its own transporter through the intestinal mucosa in the small intestine. While glucose uses the transporter SGLT-1, fructose is carried into the blood by the GLUT-5 membrane protein from the intestines in the small intestinal cells. The average person is able to absorb up to a little more than one ounce per hour of this protein; it's responsible for absorbing fructose from the intestines and releasing it into the blood, where it is then transported to the liver. For many people, however, the capacity limit is way below one ounce per hour due to hereditary or acquired reasons, such as irritable bowel syndrome, diabetes mellitus, or unfavorable composition of the intestinal flora. It is estimated that 20 percent of adults and 30 percent of children have a genetically restricted transporting function.

If there is too much fructose for the transporters to handle at once, the fructose builds up and will not be able to be absorbed. The fructose will end up in the deeper areas of the intestines and will be decomposed by intestinal bacteria. The fermenting process, in turn, will lead to typical symptoms such as bloating, flatulence, indigestion, and even diarrhea.

A limited capacity of fructose transporter GLUT-5 is clinically known as fructose malabsorption. People suffering from this are only able to absorb a certain amount of fructose per unit of time without developing problems, which will very often be misinterpreted as irritable bowel syndrome (IBS). When large amounts of glucose are eaten at the same time, the function of the fructose transporter will be stimulated and could lessen the probability of symptoms. Therefore, pure sugar (table sugar, or sucrose) is very often well tolerated by people who suffer from fructose malabsoption. However, eating sorbitol (a sugar substitute often found in chewing gum and in some fruits) in combination with fructose will often lead to problems because sorbitol competes with the same fructose transporter. The capacity limit is quickly reached and fructose will not be fully absorbed. The individual tolerance of fructose can differ from person to person. The combination of fruits you eat can also make a difference. While apples, pears, and watermelon contain a lot of fructose and less glu-

Chemical structure formulas of fruit sugar (fructose) and dextrose (glucose) and table sugar (sucrose)

cose, they typically cause more indigestion when eaten even in small amounts compared to eating fruits like bananas or apricots, which contain less fructose. Fruit juice, such as apple juice, can typically cause problems much faster than eating the actual fruit because it passes quickly through the stomach into the intestines. Even drinking .5 to .75 cups can cause discomfort.

Reactions also depend on whether the fruit is eaten on its own or as part of a meal. For example, eating an apple as a snack is more likely to cause indigestion than if eaten as a dessert, where the fructose plus the other food eaten with a meal end up in the intestines more slowly. The GLUT-5 transporter will reach its capacity levels per time unit at a slower pace, since high fat and protein-rich meals will damper the fructose.

WHAT IS FRUCTOSE?
Fructose belongs to the carbohydrate group and is considered, just as glucose, a so-called simple sugar (monosaccharide). Plants use the sweeteners of their fruits to attract animals to eat them so that their seeds can be widely distributed. Fructose is found in nearly all fruits and vegetables in different concentrations.

WHY IS FRUCTOSE SO POPULAR AMONG FOOD MANUFACTURERS?
Fructose is the sweetest of all sugars. It intensifies the taste of both sweet and savory foods. It increases the volume in pastries and gives baked goods that nice "tanned" color. It prevents harmful ice crystallization in frozen foods, is very soluble, and does not crystalize. Fructose and fructose syrup are extremely economical since they can be produced inexpensively.

HOW TO AVOID USING TOO MUCH FRUCTOSE?
- **Reduce sugar consumption:** Limit your sugar consumption consciously and consistently. Even table sugar is 50 percent fructose.
- **Avoid processed food containing fructose:** Read the ingredients list on the labels of the food you buy. Avoid all products containing fructose or fructose syrup.
- **Drink fruit juice sparingly:** Drink fruit juice—even freshly pressed/squeezed—only every once in a while. It's a lot easier to drink a cup of juice made of three or four pounds of fruit (depending on the kind of fruit juice) than eating that much fruit. It goes down a lot easier in liquid form, and so does all the fructose! And that's a lot of fructose!
- **Use honey in small quantities:** Honey usually contains more fructose than glucose and should be used sparingly. The more

liquid the honey (or better said, the longer it stays in liquid form), the more fructose content it has.
- **Eat dried fruits in small quantities:** Dried fruits are also very rich in fructose and should seldom be eaten and only in small amounts.

> **Please note!** *Apple and pear concentrated fruit juice syrups, available in many health food stores are often sold as healthy alternatives. They are, however, NOT healthy alternatives and consist mainly of fructose. For this reason, agave syrup is NOT an alternative!*

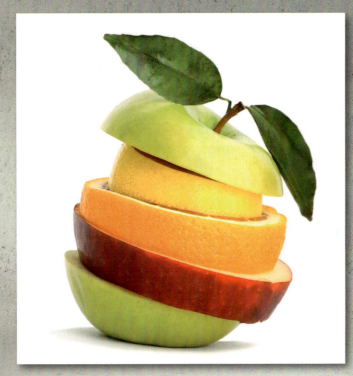

WHAT EXACTLY IS IN A FRUIT SMOOTHIE?

The term *smoothie* is an American word for a whole-fruit drink. It originated back in the 1920s in smoothie bars. A popular refreshment was a mixed drink made out of fresh-squeezed orange juice, water, egg whites, vanilla extract, sugar, and ice. It had a velvety smooth consistency.

The term smoothie as a pure fruit drink came about in the 1980s. But what exactly is in a pure fruit smoothie? And why are smoothies better than conventional juice?

It's the use of the fruit as a whole, often even including the peel, that makes smoothies healthier. Fiber and vitamins remain intact and the fructose is not in a dissolved form. Smoothies are also very satiating, which makes them a perfect replacement for breakfast or any other meal. Another advantage of smoothies compared to juice is that when drinking a smoothie, you aren't consuming an overwhelming amount of fruit.

FRUIT BELLY

"Green smoothies" are becoming the "in thing" these days. They are a mixture of fruit and vegetables and offer you the perfect opportunity to eat a nice portion of vegetables along with your fruit.

The problem with pure fruit smoothies is the fact that they are real true sugar—or better said, fructose bombs. Because there is no chewing involved, there is no pre-digestion process. When we chew our food, the digestive enzyme amylase is activated by the production of saliva, which is responsible for the digestion of carbohydrates.

It's important when making smoothies that they don't only contain carbohydrates, but also protein and fat. All smoothie recipes in this book include all of the macronutrients (fat, protein, and carbohydrates) in a balanced ratio. This will not cause blood sugar levels to rise too quickly. The pure food smoothies are easy to digest and will fill you up, in a good way, to support good digestion during the Quick Fix.

DR. ALBERS – EFFECTS OF CONSUMING TOO MUCH FRUCTOSE

By following a diet, for example the Paleo diet, where you avoid eating processed food and sugar, a fructose intake of 3/4 to 1 ounce a day is typical. However, if you eat a lot of fruit and food containing sugar (table sugar is equivalent to 50 percent fructose), fruit juice (apple and orange juice are especially highly concentrated fructose sources), you will be consuming significantly higher amounts of fructose each day. Also, the use of fructose as a sugar replacement in many foods contributes to the overconsumption of fructose in our society. The American Heart Association cites that Americans eat about 100 grams of added sugars a day according to a report from the 2005–10 NHANES (National Health and Nutrition Examination Survey) database.

Eating more than 1 to 1-3/4 ounces of sugar a day can have a negative effect on the metabolism, particularly if you are also eating too many calories, which is very common nowadays.

Because fructose is broken down differently than glucose, it also affects our metabolism differently. Fructose is metabolized in the intestines and absorbed by the liver, and is then either converted into glucose and used as a direct energy source or is stored in the form of fat for reserves. If there is already an existing energy surplus (excess calories), then the fructose will be stored as fat in the liver, which could launch the onset of long-term fatty liver disease. Nowadays, 30 to 40 percent of the population is at high risk for acquiring various diseases such as obesity, diabetes mellitus type 2, heart attacks, strokes, and kidney failure (leading to dialysis).

Accumulation of fat in the liver, such as a continuous over-supply of fructose, leads to insulin resistance of the organs, poorer blood-fat levels (increased levels of triglycerides and decreased levels of the "good" HDL cholesterol), and poorer blood sugar levels. This in turn promotes blood sugar swings, cravings, and hunger attacks, which then result in binging (increased calorie intake), especially on foods high in sugar and carbohydrates. Fructose, in comparison to glucose, has a less satiating effect that will cause us to want more and more to be satisfied. A fatty liver combined with excess calories in the form of unhealthy, sugar-rich foods causes a vicious cycle that will only get worse with time. In the long run, we will only end up getting sick, potentially developing diabetes. Not only will the liver be affected, but excess energy will also be stored in subcutaneous and abdominal fat.

Thus, a high intake of fructose over a long period of time not only increases subcutaneous and abdominal fat, but also causes a range of negative effects on the metabolism because of a high-fructose induced fatty liver. Poor cholesterol levels, poor blood sugar metabolism (leading to diabetes mellitus type 2), and damage to blood vessels leading to accelerated atherosclerosis (hardening of the arteries) could result in high health risks such as heart attack and stroke—which in America and other western countries are the main cause of death.

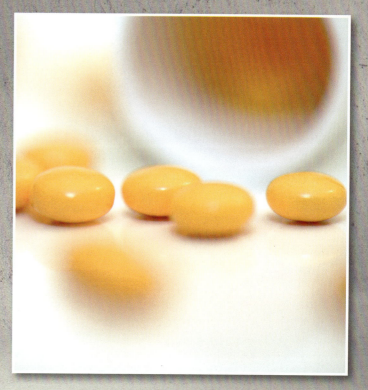

DR. ALBERS – HOW IS FRUCTOSE INTOLERANCE DETECTED?

The safest and most reliable test to detect fructose intolerance is known as the hydrogen breath test. The patient drinks a solution of ¾ ounce of pure fructose in ¾ cup of water on an empty stomach. The hydrogen levels are measured by blowing into a special device (similar to the one used when taking an alcohol test) every 30 minutes over a two-hour period. Usually in healthy people, after drinking the fructose solution, hydrogen concentration levels are under 20 ppm (parts per million). That's less than 0.0020 percent. If the levels are higher during the two-hour test, this could indicate that hydrogen gas is being produced in the intestines. This happens when bacteria ferment the undigested fructose in the large intestine. Hydrogen is released into the bloodstream from the intestinal mucosa and is then exhaled through the lungs. If the small intestines are easily able to absorb the amount of fructose taken in the test (equivalent to approximately two large apples), that fructose will not be fermented by bacteria in the large intestine and there will be no sign of hydrogen in the exhaled air. Thus, the hydrogen breath test will be negative at normal intestinal absorption.

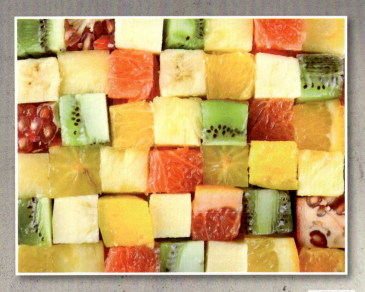

THE TRANSFORMATION OF FRUITS

The earliest apples were much smaller than the ones we find in the supermarkets today. They had a maximal diameter of 1.2 inches. Compared to the sweet and juicy apple varieties of today, the ancient apples tasted very sour due to their tannin content. However, everyone has their preference: there are now thousands of different kinds of apples exported all over the world. The ones we find at the grocery store are just a small "taste" of what's out there.

It's no different with strawberries: strawberry farms grow five to six different kinds of strawberries every year. But they have lost their original taste and flavor. Scientists believe that the original strawberry had a slightly bitter taste, but was still delicious. Obviously, the strategy nowadays is to produce the most beautiful, big, red, disease-resistant strawberries possible, and not focus on the actual taste of the fruit. Since fruit often has to be transported long distances, it has to be durable and look good, since this is what the buyer wants and expects. Today's strawberries may be tempting—large, ruby red, perfectly packed in little containers—but when you bite into them, you're very often disappointed with the bland, watery taste in your mouth. The flavors have been lost over the years due to over-breeding.

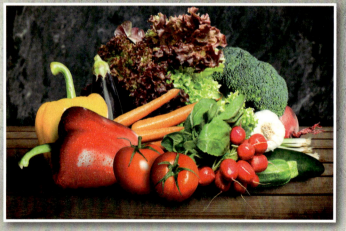

IN A DIET WITHOUT FRUIT, DO WE GET ENOUGH VITAMINS?

We all know that fruit is healthy. We have to eat fruit to get enough vitamins. We must eat two servings of fruit and three servings of vegetables each day. We don't get enough vitamins if we don't eat our fruits and vegetables.

Well, these statements aren't necessarily false, except for the last one. You can cover your daily vitamin requirement very easily without fruit. Organically grown, fully ripened fruits are a wonderful source of vitamins, but we are not dependent on them. As long as we increase the amounts of vegetables we eat, we are not at risk of insufficient vitamin intake. If you suspect probable fructose intolerance, the only way to allow your body to recover is by limiting your intake of fructose. Very often, vegetables are even more nutrient dense than fruit.

Many of us have it in our heads that fruit for breakfast or as a snack is the way to go, and could never imagine eating cauliflower, for example, for breakfast. It's all in the way we look at it, and much of the time, it's a matter of habit.

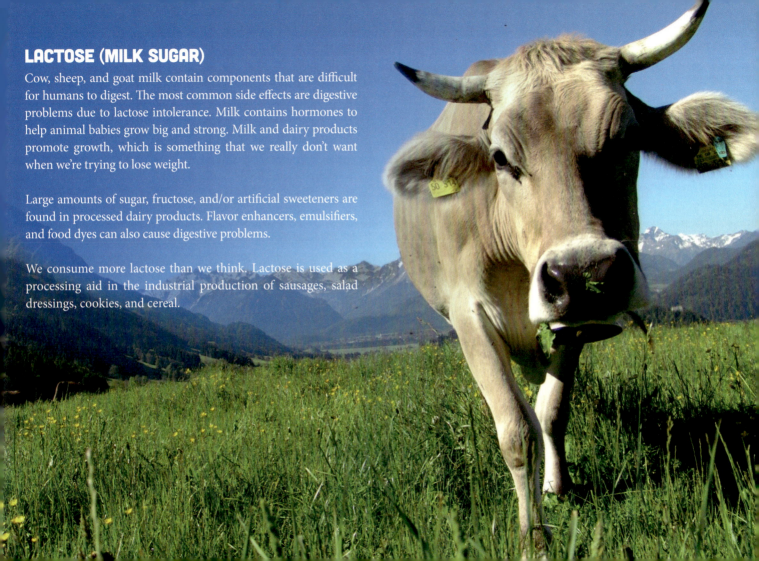

LACTOSE (MILK SUGAR)

Cow, sheep, and goat milk contain components that are difficult for humans to digest. The most common side effects are digestive problems due to lactose intolerance. Milk contains hormones to help animal babies grow big and strong. Milk and dairy products promote growth, which is something that we really don't want when we're trying to lose weight.

Large amounts of sugar, fructose, and/or artificial sweeteners are found in processed dairy products. Flavor enhancers, emulsifiers, and food dyes can also cause digestive problems.

We consume more lactose than we think. Lactose is used as a processing aid in the industrial production of sausages, salad dressings, cookies, and cereal.

> **What is lactose?**
> Lactose refers to the sugar naturally found in milk produced by mammals. It is found in cow milk, sheep milk, goat milk, mare milk, and of course in human breast milk. The average lactose content is anywhere between 2 and 7 percent. Lactose belongs to the twofold sugars, consisting of glucose and galactose. In order for the body to be able to use this twofold sugar as energy, it must first be split into two components. Our body does this by using the enzyme lactase.

Diarrhea is also a symptom of lactose intolerance. This is an efficient way for the body to cleanse itself, by flushing the intestines. This is probably the most common and uncomfortable symptom of lactose intolerance. The symptoms usually begin within a few hours after consuming lactose.

WHAT IS LACTOSE INTOLERANCE?

Lactose intolerance is not a disease or an allergy—it's a food intolerance. This is not to be confused with milk protein allergy. The reason for lactose intolerance is the complete absence or insufficient production of the body's digestive enzyme lactase. The enzyme lactase is found in the small intestine and splits the twofold sugar lactose into its two components, glucose and galactose, since only simple sugars can be absorbed by the intestines.

If there is a lack of lactase or insufficient lactase activity, the un-split lactose will end up in the large intestine where it will be fermented by intestinal bacteria. This, in turn, will lead to discomfort such as cramps, bloating, and flatulence. Since these gases are also exhaled, the hydrogen breath test can be used to diagnose lactose intolerance.

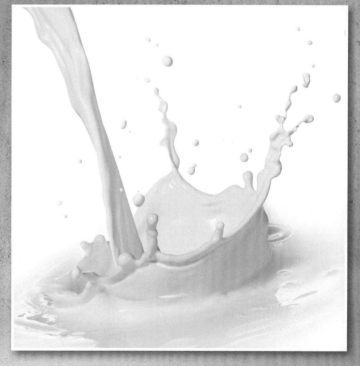

SYMPTOMS OF LACTOSE INTOLERANCE:

- Stomachache
- Cramps
- Bloating
- Feeling full
- Vomiting
- Constipation
- Diarrhea

The symptoms will increase with the amount of lactose consumed. The symptoms seem to be worse if lactose intolerance is caused by genetic conditions rather than acquiring it later in life due to a decrease of lactase production, which is common as we get older.

WHY IS THERE LACTOSE IN PACKED DELI-STYLE COOKED HAM?

Here's an explanation for why you can find lactose in ham and why it is used in food production. Maybe you've decided to avoid lactose and add a bit more meat into your diet. Well, if you think you can eat as much ham and salami as you want, you are going to be disappointed. Because salami is a processed meat, it really doesn't belong on your plate. The same goes for other deli-style meats, such as cooked ham, dried beef or ham, and cured or smoked ham. Because of its water-binding ability, lactose is often used as a binder by the food industry and also by the pharmaceutical industry. In addition, by adding lactose to food, the food manufacturers are able to achieve a higher food density, volume, and weight, without adding more calories. This is why it is used in many "light," reduced-calorie products, in addition to packaged meat. Lactose also acts as a flavor enhancer.

Conclusion: please check ingredients labels, even of the products you have always bought in the past. Better to be safe than sorry.

YOGURT: IS IT GOOD FOR YOU AND YOUR DIGESTION?

We hear and read every day about how healthy yogurt is. Unfortunately, this is not true for the most part. Conventional yogurts contain lactose (milk sugar) and casein (milk protein), which can cause negative reactions. Many people are also intolerant. Flavored yogurts are filled with additives (artificial flavoring, artificial sweeteners, fructose, stabilizers). Our body recognizes these additives as foreign substances and becomes confused. "Light" or reduced-fat yogurts cause blood sugar levels to rise and make it difficult for the body to burn body fat. They actually do the exact opposite of what the food manufacturers promise in their advertisements.

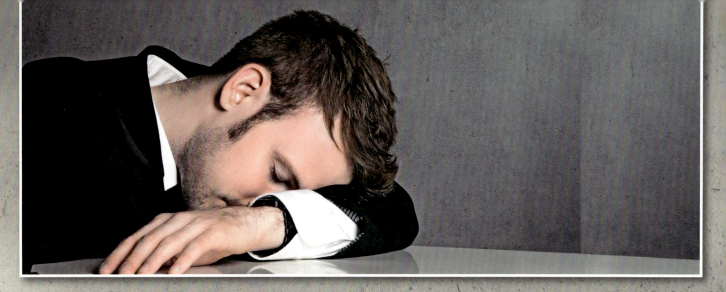

These additives not only make it extremely difficult or even impossible to lose weight, they also promote the growth of bad intestinal bacteria and fungus. In addition, all industrially produced yogurts are pasteurized and homogenized. So you are pretty much consuming dead food. All the beneficial bacteria that promote good digestion have been killed.

If industrial yogurt is produced with milk from cows that were treated with antibiotics, then we will also be getting a dose of those antibiotics. Not to mention the hormones that milk contains, even if the cows were not treated with hormones. Hormones are still found in milk even after pasteurization and homogenization. This can have a negative effect on our own hormones when we eat yogurt. It could very well be that "healthy" yogurt can cause more harm than good: bloating, flatulence, acne, headaches, constipation, brain fog, candida, eczema, irregular or painful menstruation, and disturbances in hormonal balance.

If you can't resist the temptation of creamy yogurt, then stick to kinds that are organic and free of additives—read the ingredients. Or you could make your own. However, if you are intolerant or sensitive to lactose or casein, even the purest natural yogurt can cause problems.

DR. ALBERS – NOT ENOUGH CALCIUM WITHOUT DAIRY PRODUCTS?

Calcium has multiple functions in our bodies: it is responsible for contracting muscles and helping blood clot, and is an important enzyme component that is a building block for bones and teeth. We often think that enough calcium equals healthy bones. However, healthy bones and sufficient bone density are not only dependent on the amount of calcium we ingest, but also on an optimized diet and lifestyle, especially as we get older. This includes primarily getting enough physical activity (especially weight training), sunshine (vitamin D), vitamin K, and magnesium, as well as limiting your intake of phosphate (soft drinks, processed foods and meats) and regulating your stress levels. A high intake of calcium without enough exercise and vitamin D will most likely lead to premature bone loss over the course of aging, just as eating a lot of protein will not promote muscle growth without training.

There are many other natural sources of calcium besides dairy products. Calcium is also found in nuts (such as almonds, hazelnuts, and walnuts), kale, spinach, bok choy, broccoli, amaranth (botanically broadly known as a grain), oats, and seeds (flaxseed and sesame seeds).

HISTAMINE INTOLERANCE

The symptoms of histaminosis (histamine intolerance) are similar to those of an allergy, food poisoning, or a cold. They are very often triggered by eating a certain food, but they can also be chronic or can intermittently emerge without a clear connection with a food. The range of unspecific symptoms is enormously wide. The symptoms will differ from person to person. Typical symptoms could be:

- Nasal congestion, runny nose, sneezing, coughing, difficulty breathing
- Digestive problems: diarrhea, stomachaches, bloating, heartburn
- Itching, rashes, hives, redness of the skin, flushed face (red cheeks)
- Hot flashes, sudden sweating, temperature sensitivity
- Cardiac arrhythmia (accelerated heart rate)
- Hypotension (drop in blood pressure)
- Headaches, migraines, dizziness
- Sleep disorders, fatigue
- Nausea, vomiting
- Irregular menstrual cycles
- Edema (tissue swelling, such as swollen eyelids)

Acute or chronic gastrointestinal problems are frequent symptoms of histaminosis. There could be many reasons for these unspecific problems, often referred to as dyspepsia or IBS. It's difficult to determine whether there is a direct connection to the food we eat, since it sometimes takes hours for the food to be digested, metabolized, and make its way to the intestines.

Common complaints include chronic diarrhea or regular morning diarrhea, since histamine increases gastrointestinal motility, which then causes food to pass through the body faster than normal. Since the food is only in the intestines for a short period of time, it is not properly digested. Constipation or a combination of diarrhea and constipation is a less frequent symptom.

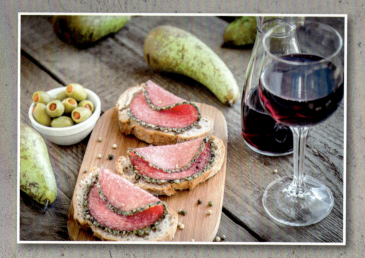

What is histamine?
Histamine is a messenger chemical that controls many functions. It is a signal transmitter, alerting the body in cases of infection and allergic reactions. It is an infection mediator, tissue hormone, and neurotransmitter. It influences the sleep-wake state, intestinal movements, and many other operations. Histamine is produced in the body and stored in mast cells and other specialized cell types, and when necessary, is immediately released. Especially in allergic reactions (overreacting of the immune system), histamine will be released in large amounts, which in turn will lead to allergic symptoms. Histamine can also be externally supplied directly through the food we eat, or can be produced by the intestinal flora. Histamine is a fermentation, maturation, or deterioration product found in most foods at different levels of concentration. Perishable products are mostly histamine-free when fresh, but can turn into real "histamine bombs" if stored for long periods of time. Large amounts of histamine are found in conserved and preserved fish, cured and dried meats, aged cheese, wine, champagne, beer, vinegar, and in other fermented products. Also, the intestinal flora will produce histamine, especially when there is an overgrowth of harmful microorganisms (dysbiosis).

WHAT IS HISTAMINE INTOLERANCE (HISTAMINOSIS)?

Histamine intolerance is characterized by an impairment of the well-being and normal physical/mental functions of the body as a result of abnormal levels of histamine.

Influenced by a number of factors, histamine is produced naturally by the body and is released from the storage cells; it can also be supplied from external sources. If, for whatever reason, histamine levels exceed the body's ability to break it down, histamine levels will become too high. There are many reasons for this. An enzymatic histamine metabolic disorder is called histamine intolerance. However, clinical relevance is still controversial and the lack of meaningful methods of diagnosis makes it difficult to find the reason for abnormal histamine levels. Unfavorable environmental influences have an effect on the physical causes of difficulty in breaking down histamine. Dietary habits, taking incompatible medications, environmental toxins, and stress can also influence histamine levels.

Histamine intolerance is therefore not an allergy, but a poisoning by a messenger substance that makes the body unable to hold on to the set point. This condition is not just influenced by food intolerance, but also by many other factors. Besides physical causes, behavior and environment determine whether and how much you are affected. It is possible that there are a number of causes that lead to this serious disease.

It is assumed that two percent of the population is affected, but there are no exact numbers. Women are affected more often than men.

HOW CAN I RECOGNIZE HISTAMINE INTOLERANCE?

The only reliable diagnosis known is by completing a multi-week elimination diet, which cuts out all foods that could cause histamine problems. The patients are clearly instructed on how to do this and are recommended to keep a food/health problem diary.

If after the first few days there is a noticeable improvement of symptoms, then you could suspect histaminosis. Subsequently, the patient should be able to determine his individual tolerance by slowly introducing, step by step, the avoided food and observe the reactions.

Histaminosis can be treated by following a histamine elimination diet (reducing or eliminating histamine trigger foods). Additionally, the therapy can be supported with medicine and food supplements. Living a stress-free lifestyle can have a positive effect also. It's important for people suffering from allergies to avoid allergens.

WHAT KINDS OF FOOD CONTAINS HISTAMINE?

Histamine rich foods are foods that have undergone fermentation, maturation, or long-term storage: spoiled fish, conserved fish, sausage and dried meat, aged cheese, wine, champagne, beer, vinegar, and other fermented products. Since histamine is heat and cold resistant, it cannot be removed by cooking or freezing the food.

Other foods to avoid are sauerkraut, spinach, tomatoes, eggplant, avocado, legumes (lentils, beans, soy), strawberries, raspberries, citrus, bananas, pineapples, kiwi, pears, papaya, nuts, many spices, and certain food additives. It's best to prepare your meals using fresh, unprocessed, raw food and consume it quickly or freeze immediately.

INDIGESTION WITH RAW FOOD

Have you ever felt bloated and not well after eating a big salad or a bowl of fruit? Do you have phases when you can tolerate raw food better than others?

Do you feel overwhelmed by so-called dietary guidelines and alternative healing methods because you don't know what's good for you or what to believe anymore?

In the next section, you'll find your answers. You will learn the meaning of "raw food," how your digestive system works and reacts to raw food, and how other alternative healing methods such as Traditional Chinese Medicine (TCM) and Ayurveda stand on raw food.

WHAT IS RAW FOOD?

Raw food is generally perceived as a vegetarian diet consisting of primarily raw vegetables. But as it happens, foods such as honey, cold pressed oils, dried fruits or dried meat are also included. The raw food diet could be vegetarian (lacto-vegetable diet) or purely vegan, but it could also just mean raw food, which would include a variety of animal products as long as they were not treated with heat. So all kinds of fruits, vegetables, herbs, olives, nuts, seeds, mushrooms and untreated oils are included in the raw food range. Also, all raw milk products belong on the list, assuming that you are not following a vegan raw food diet. Raw meat and fish would be allowed on a (non vegetarian/vegan) raw food diet: raw meat (beef tartar), cured and smoked meat, fish (smoked salmon), and tuna fish (sashimi).

THE DARK SIDE OF RAW FOOD

Perhaps you are among the many people who believe that eating salads and raw foods will help you lose weight. Maybe you've even tried eating a raw food diet and wondered why your belly became even bigger. You may now understand that it was gas in your belly making you so bloated. This gas is produced when proteins decompose and carbohydrates ferment. Salad, vegetables, and fruit are also fermenting-friendly foods. While fermenting, toxic alcohol is formed, which is more difficult for your body to metabolize than a glass of wine. This also contributes to over acidification in your body. Consequently, this leads to the uncomfortable bloated feeling from a gas-filled belly. And if you also feel tired and irritable, this is clearly a sign of an irritable nervous system.

However, there are people who can easily tolerate a raw food diet. This is because each of us has a "unique genetic code:" an individual metabolism and unique intestinal flora. The differences are measured by the acidity of the stomach, the length of the intestines, the active role of genetics, and the functionality of digestion and detoxification enzymes. The right diet is therefore highly individual and often culturally dependent.

DIGESTIVE POWER

By eating and drinking, our body is supplied with power (energy) and the building material for the formation of new cells. Our digestive system has the following functions: it processes food so that it can be absorbed by the body, regulates nutrient intake, and eliminates non-digested food particles. In addition, the intestines play a big role in isolating microorganisms and intestinal flora. For this reason, the majority of immune competent cells are found in the intestines.

WHAT HAPPENS TO THE FOOD THAT YOU EAT?

Digestion already begins in your mouth; when you chew your food, your salivary glands secrete a fluid that contains the digestive enzyme amylase, among others. This enzyme breaks down carbohydrates into sugar units, which is the reason why bread acquires a sweet taste if chewed long enough. In situations of stress, saliva production is reduced and will cause you to have a dry mouth. Therefore, digestive problems can already begin in your mouth in times of stress and will later move on to your stomach.

The function of your stomach isn't just to collect food, it also plays an important digestive role. Protein and fat are broken down (with pepsin and lipases) and are predigested. Stomach acid is responsible for killing most bacteria ingested with the food, destroys protein-containing allergens, and prevents allergies. These are very important properties that are unfortunately destroyed by acid blockers and antacids (stomach acid binding agents).

The stomach then transports only enough food that the intestines are able to break down. If the stomach empties too quickly or too slowly, unpleasant symptoms could develop.

The small and large intestines are considered the most important digestive stations. However, their roles are completely different.

THE SMALL INTESTINE

The small intestine usually contains just a small number of bacteria, about 100 to a maximum of 100,000 per mL of intestinal content. The gallbladder and the pancreas secrete digestive fluid into the small intestine, breaking down fat, carbohydrates, and protein into nutrients. So-called "pumps" in the intestinal wall transport the nutrients from the intestines into the lymph and bloodstream. These building blocks are necessary for the body's metabolism. This process is called resorption. If there are disorders present in the gallbladder or pancreas, digestive problems could arise. If there are substances that can't be broken down or transported through the small intestine, they are moved on to the large intestine as dietary fiber. It is often these food components that promote food intolerances.

THE LARGE INTESTINE

Undigested food or dietary fiber is converted through the process of fermentation by intestinal bacteria in the large intestine. Bacterial by-products are transformed into useful substances or detoxified. Gas is produced in this process and is often noticeable as flatulence. A large amount of food particles in the large intestine leads to increased gas formation. At the same time, the fermentation process produces short-chained fatty acids, which in turn draws water into the large intestine, which could result in diarrhea.

In the rectum, as much water as possible is withdrawn from the stool so that it will have a thicker consistency.

THE DIFFERENCE BETWEEN DISGESTION IN MEN AND WOMEN

Women tend to struggle with indigestion over twice as much as men do. More than two thirds of people suffering from digestive problems are women. Some of the problems include indigestion and constipation. Gynecologists have come to the conclusion that there is a connection between digestion and female hormones. It has been found that women are particularly affected with digestive issues due to hormonal changes, such as during menstruation, pregnancy or menopause. This suggests that female sex hormones have an indirect impact on the digestive system. Estrogen and progesterone have a big influence on the gastrointestinal tract. Serotonin also plays a large part in this. Surprisingly, about 95 percent of this tissue hormone is active in the intestines and not, as expected, in the brain. It is responsible for different digestive functions in the intestines, mainly

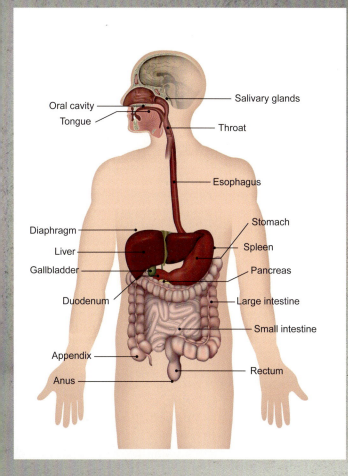

the flexibility of the intestines. Estrogen has a positive effect on serotonin. Serotonin receptors are increased and become more sensitively responsive. In the brain, serotonin is responsible for creating a better mood, and in the intestines, it promotes functional intestinal movement. Estrogen also provides a better flow of bile so that the chyme (partly digested food) is easily digested. However, if progesterone is increased, this will weaken the effects of serotonin.

Progesterone levels rise in the second half of the menstrual cycle. Under the influence of progesterone, the intestinal movement becomes sluggish, the serotonin activity at the receptors is at a low, and the bile flow is reduced. Studies have shown that during the progesterone phase, the transitional time (the period from eating the food to the excretion) takes considerably longer. This is the reason many women experience constipation during this time of the month.

Many hormonal changes occur when a woman reaches her mid-forties or enters menopause. This process normally lasts 10 to 15 years. During this time, estrogen production is reduced and the serotonin signal transmitters to intestinal receptors are impaired. This contributes to a slower digestion.

CHAPTER 3 | REASONS FOR HAVING A FAT BELLY

WHAT WEAKENS THE DIGESTIVE POWER?

Digestion is weakened by improper diet (like too much salad and fruit), stress, poor composition of intestinal bacteria, disease, food intolerance... the list goes on.

HOW DO TRADITIONAL CHINESE MEDICINE AND AYURVEDA STAND ON RAW FOOD?

Traditional Chinese Medicine (TCM) and Ayurveda are two philosophical systems that are characterized by an extensive healing knowledge on the subject of health. Raw food is not recommended by either of the two, in particular TCM, because high digestive power is needed when breaking down raw foods.

Digestive problems, especially caused by raw foods, indicate a weakened Spleen Qi. Symptoms include fatigue, cravings for sweets, loose stools, a susceptibility to fungal infections, edema, and frequent colds. TCM describes the digestion as the "root of health." Stomach rumbling, problems such as bloating, heartburn, stomachaches and/or alternating loose stools indicate an imbalance in the body. Both teachings emphasize that food can trigger constructive and also destructive effects in the body. Food can be used as a "pick-me-up", a regeneration of the body or assistance in being more active, but it can also have a complete opposite effect. Both teachings point out that not every food is good for everyone. What is good for you could cause bloating in another person. This is why it is extremely important to find out what's good for you, your body, your mind, and your soul.

EMOTIONAL INFLUENCES

Today I'm going to treat myself. I had a stressful day, which allows me to shamelessly grab some of that chocolate in the refrigerator, enjoy some cookies from the cookie jar or chips while sitting in front of the TV. And, without a guilty conscience, because today I deserve it! How satisfying it is to have a piece of chocolate slowly melt on your tongue or to lick the salt from your lips and indulge in the intoxication of happy hormones? Does this sound like a reward? Maybe you've ignored your cravings all day or you didn't have time to eat. After a long day at work, you want to give in to your cravings and desires and pursue your longing for gratification—to lose control and reach for the food that triggers feelings of happiness.

We not only search for that feeling of happiness on a daily basis, but our whole life long. We go on diets to attain our dream figure so that we can be happy with our dream body. We work overtime to afford and find happiness in our house in the country. We work on the weekends to save up for our dream vacation so that we'll be happy on the beach under the palm trees. The pursuit of happiness dominates us, each of us in its own way. Therefore it is not at all surprising that we want to reward ourselves at the end of the day with something that

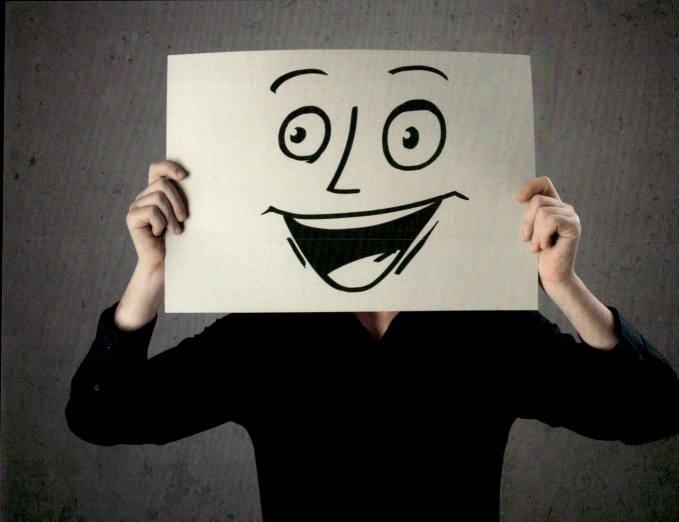

triggers feelings of happiness. The neural reward system in our brain gives the orders.

If the reward is in sight, our brain is motivated to act. The neural reward system is a system of neurons that uses dopamine as a neurotransmitter. These neurotransmitters are involved in the development of positive feelings. How does the reward system work? Desire arises in the cerebral cortex. If you give in to your desire, signals are sent to the limbic system and to the hippocampus—then back again to the cerebral cortex: the feedback that the desire was satisfied arrives.

THE DIFFERENCE BETWEEN PHYSICAL AND EMOTIONAL HUNGER

Emotions with food. Not only the basic requirements of life such as hunger and thirst force us to behave the way we do, but also feelings of joy, sadness, stress or loneliness can lead us to the temptation of eating. If the requirement is met, then a feeling of happiness is the reward. The boundaries of consciousness and the subconscious lie close together. Am I eating because I can consciously feel the need to eat (hunger), or am I eating because I want to subconsciously activate the reward system to get rid of a bad feeling? People should once more learn to eat consciously, only when there is a noticeable feeling of hunger present. However, how do we know that this hunger is real?

Hunger is not controlled by the stomach. Even if you didn't have a stomach you could still feel hungry. If your stomach growls, it's not speaking to let you know it's empty. Your enteric nervous system is responsible for this. The enteric nervous system is in control of contracting the muscles of the gastrointestinal tract. The esophagus, stomach, and intestines contract and expand: this keeps the digestive tract clean. Since the system is always in motion, even a full stomach can make growling noises. So even if your stomach is growling, this is not an indication of "real hunger." Hunger and satiety are steered by hormones. The hunger center in the hypothalamus (dual center hypothesis) also plays a big roll: it is here that hunger and satiety feelings are controlled. If blood sugar levels are low, it becomes active. The adrenal glands are then activated to release the stress hormone adrenaline and send the person on a mission to find food. If there is no food available, the brain will turn to the glucose reserves. Since glucose is not able to get into the muscles without insulin, the brain will order the body to stop releasing it. Since the brain will hoard all the glucose, the muscles have to manage without any glucose. Metabolism is manipulated in favor of the brain. If there is still no food supplied, the body will turn to the protein reserves (muscles) in order to supply itself with energy.

Besides these neurological processes, one's emotional background also plays a big role. Emotional factors often cause a subconscious craving for food, and are connected to feelings of happiness. It is extremely difficult to distinguish if I'm really hungry or if I simply have the desire to eat something because I associate that food with feelings of happiness. For example, hunger for love may be satisfied with food. According to nutritional scientist Uwe Knop, many people have forgotten how to listen to their true biological hunger. Although according to a survey, 76 percent of respondents said that they really know their real hunger. But the fact is, hunger and satiety are complex, and hunger and appetite are not easily differentiated. Uwe Knop notes a clear difference between biological hunger and compensatory eating, where the soul is fed. He recommends getting to know these two feelings and learn their differences.

We also eat and drink when we are not physically hungry:

- Out of spite
- As a means of distraction
- Out of habit (because it's lunch time)
- Traditional customs (birthday cake or Christmas cookies)
- Out of boredom
- Opportunity (there's a bowl of candy on the table)
- Out of politeness (Mom baked something especially for me)
- Peer pressure (all my friends are drinking a beer)
- Stress (when we very often crave sweet and fatty foods)

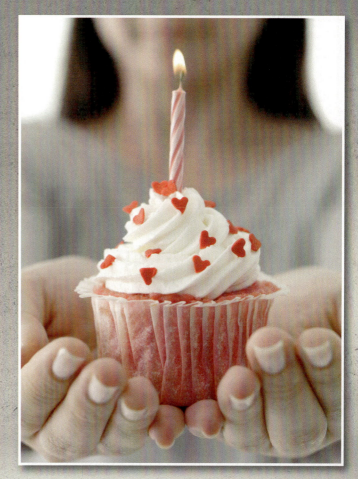

CHAPTER 3 | REASONS FOR HAVING A FAT BELLY

STRESS

The heart is racing, the stomach is cramped, the shoulder muscles are tensed, and your body is pushing for one thing: fight or flight! Everyone experiences situations that trigger feelings of stress. Family conflicts, lack of sleep, health issues, busy schedules, traffic jams or financial problem are just a few situations that allow stress hormones to skyrocket. In some situations, the head is able to react quickly—automatically analyzing and evaluating based on previous experiences. If you've experienced the same situation in the past and were able to cope, then it will seem less overwhelming this time around. You experience stress when you are not sure if you can cope with the current situation. Thoughts and feelings play a big roll. Preprogramming the situation already by saying or thinking "I can't do this!" or "I'm lost!" can create physical reactions such as rapid breathing, muscle tension, increased blood pressure, etc.

Stress is an activation reaction of the body. Whether the activation is harmful or beneficial to your health, depends solely on how you judge the stress factors. There are situations that are very stressful for everyone, such as unemployment, serious diseases, or when a family member has had an accident. But mostly it's minor situations that stress us out in our daily lives, like being being stuck in a traffic jam. How you manage this depends on your individual strategies. However, the physical reactions are the same for everyone. If you think the situation is life threatening, your body with

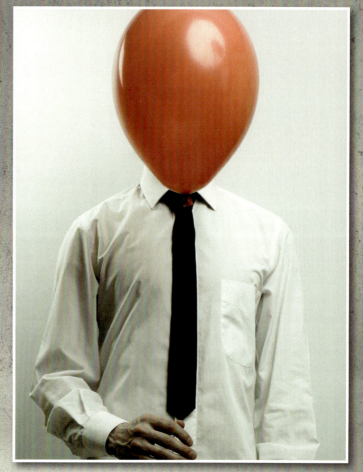

FRUIT BELLY

gather all its strength and stress hormones are released to provide you with the energy to either "fight or flight."

In the earlier history of mankind, as in the Stone Age, this mechanism was very beneficial. It ensured survival. This was the only way it was possible to run away from a wild animal or other dangerous situations. Even today, there are situations in which we find this mechanism to be to our advantage. In dangerous situations, our body reacts automatically, without having to think about our actions. Thinking and analyzing would surely be a waste of time, which explains why we sometimes experience mental blocks in stressful situations. But in other certain situations, is it possible to control this burst of energy and relax? What exactly happens? You become psychologically alert, internal pressure continues to build up, and that built-up energy works against your body. Short stressful situations like these are manageable and you are able to relax relatively quickly. Chronic stress, however, is a completely different picture.

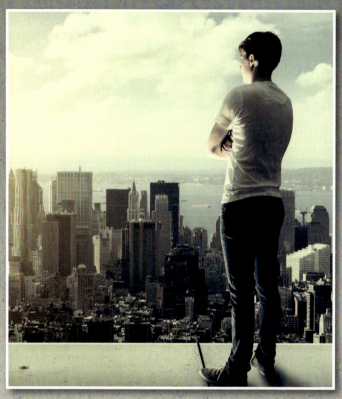

CHRONIC STRESS MAKES YOU FAT
With chronic stress your body is constantly on alert and there is no physical or mental balance. This leads to permanent exhaustion, which will in turn promote disease. Many people tend to gain weight when under a constant state of chronic stress. Scientists at Ohio State University (OSU) have studied this tendency and researched the causes. They tested insulin and blood sugar levels, blood lipid levels, and cortisol levels in a group of healthy women before and after eating. Some of the women were exposed to various stressful situations within 24 hours before the testing. It appears that the body burns fewer calories when exposed to

stress. In addition, insulin levels were higher in the women that were exposed to stress compared to the group not exposed. Elevated levels of insulin block the conversion of fat into energy, leading to insufficient fat loss. As a result, more fat is stored in the tissue, suggesting a long-term increase of body weight.

A study found that chronic stress causes belly fat to accumulate more and faster than a diet high in sugar. Stress also encourages high blood pressure, infections, high cholesterol levels, glucose intolerance, cardiovascular disease, and diabetes.

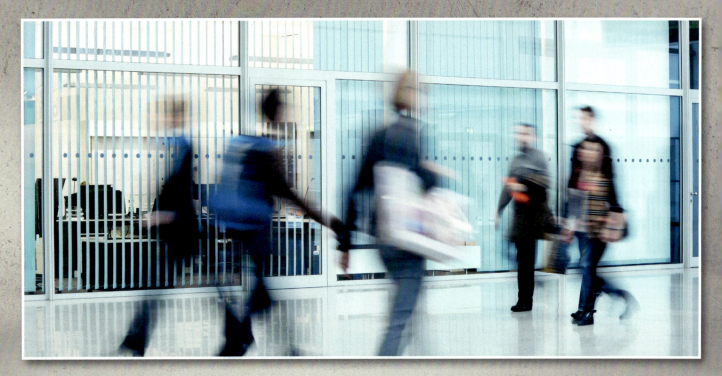

Posture-Breathing-Digestion

Taking a deep breath, inhaling and exhaling. Why should this be good for my belly? This will make my belly stick out even more while inhaling! That's exactly the way it should be!

The connection between posture, breathing, and digestion is not widely known. Our breathing is "controlled" by our diaphragm. When inhaling, the diaphragm is pushed down into the abdominal cavity and into the organs. The stomach is pushed out and air is drawn into the lungs. When exhaling, the diaphragm is pushed up again, the stomach retracts, and air is pressed out of the lungs.

This all appears very forced and tiring. But our body is so sophisticated that it does everything automatically, as all of our bodily functions are aligned accordingly. Our intestines and our digestion are dependent on this "massage" by the diaphragm. If our body doesn't get this "massage" caused by the simple act of breathing, we get indigestion, which leads to flatulence and bloating.

An estimated 50 percent of all people chronically hyperventilate, meaning that they are only breathing into their chest area over long periods of time. This puts the body into a chronic state of stress. (Our bodies are designed to supply oxygen in times of stress to the muscles, not to the brain, and especially not to the digestion system—we can think and digest later, after the stress has gone.)

Our posture is the basic prerequisite that allows the process of breathing to take place. Having bent or curved posture, such as while sitting, prevents the ability to inhale deeply. Here's a very effective exercise you can do:

- Sit upright, comfortably on a chair. Your breathing is a relaxed abdominal breathing (normal breathing)
- Now make a frown. What happens to your breathing? Yes, you'll suddenly breath only into your chest.
- Now pull your shoulders up to your ears then let them drop, relax your face muscles and let go of that frown. What happens? Exactly, you are once again able, to breath into your abdomen.

It's no wonder why people who sit at their desks all day on the computer and don't get any physical activity, and pay no attention to their posture and breathing, will very often suffer from bloating and indigestion in the evenings, no matter what they ate that day. And this in return will cause more stress, leading to once again breathing only into your chest.

If you are relaxed, have good posture, and breath evenly, you can create circumstances in which that your digestion can run smoothly. And you didn't even have to look at what was on your plate today. Therefore—practice good posture while sitting or walking, breath deeply into the abdomen, relax your face muscles, and allow your shoulders to relax. Doing this before you eat is even more important, because if you are relaxed, you can properly digest your food.

EXERCISE

Do you have a big belly even though you do a lot of sports? Do you go for hour-long jogs and still disappointed that your belly just won't go away? Or is it difficult for you to get motivated to do sports because your couch seems way more comfortable in the evenings after a long day? Is going to the gym not an option because you really don't want to become a muscle man/woman anyway?

MUSCLES—EFFECTIVE AGAINST FAT AND WEIGHT PROBLEMS

The organ with the highest energy consumption is the muscle. You have 500 skeletal muscles that are just waiting for movement and circulation. Did you know that well trained muscles, either active or not, require far more energy than untrained muscles? This means that people who work out on a regular basis (two to three times a week) will in the long run have a faster metabolism.

STRENGTH TRAINING MAKES MUSCLES INTO FAT BURNING MACHINES

One single strength training session will increase the metabolism for 48 hours. On the other hand, this positive effect will only last for half an hour after a cardio training session. A study at University of Wisconsin found that it is possible to specifically shape the body by strength training. For example, a woman is able to gain 2 to 4 pounds muscle mass during her first year of training. A positive side effect is simultaneous fat loss. Men are able to gain 9 to 11 pounds muscle mass within the first year due to higher testosterone levels, which leads to gaining muscle and losing fat even faster. In both men and women, noticeable success was achieved within the first three months.

THE WOMAN PHENOMENON—"THE FEAR OF MUSCLES"

Women are more hesitant when it comes to working out on machines or training with weights because they have a fear of becoming a "muscle woman." But there is no need for fear. In most women, muscle tissue accumulates quite quickly. This increased muscle tension is disproportioned in the first three months. The circulation improves and the body has a noticeable "pumped-up" effect. At this point, many women panic because their jeans may be a bit tighter than before. But in reality, muscles react quicker than the actual burning of fat. If you stop training at this point, there is a chance of tissue tension loss. Normally the circumference, let's say on the legs, will be reduced because active muscles will also burn more fat. Conclusion: the more muscle mass you have, the more fat you will burn!

When addressing an inability to gain muscle and an expansion of the belly, women should take the following points into consideration:

- Not training intensively enough
- Not strength training or not using heavy enough weights
- Too much endurance training

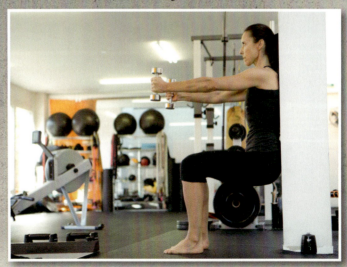

CHAPTER 3 | REASONS FOR HAVING A FAT BELLY

> **Targeted Fat Loss**
>
> Another misconception that still lurks in the minds of people is the assumption that targeted fat loss is possible. You can do as many abdominal exercises as you'd like, your belly fat will not go away with this alone. The body doesn't turn to specific areas of fat reserves for energy, but to all its fat reserves. There will be no significant fat loss when you only train single, usually small, muscles because the body is not challenged enough. Unfortunately, people think they can do crunches and sit-ups to lose belly fat, but unfortunately in this case only the opposite effect will be achieved. It is true that abdominal exercises work the abdominal muscles, but these exercises do not burn fat. In fact, the fat will remain and your belly appear even bigger, as the newly trained abdominal muscles beneath will push the fat out even farther.

REST AND RELAXATION

In order to perform efficiently long-term, you have to treat yourself to breaks. Finding time to relax, even in a busy day, is not that difficult. Everyone has to find what works best for them to reduce the stress in their life—be it sports, yoga, fitness, reading, or meditating. The latter allows you to focus on your breathing and especially helps you find serenity and inner peace. If you find yourself in a stressful situation, try to focus on your breathing and slow it down. This will distract you from what's stressing you out and will calm you down quickly. In order to really calm yourself, it's necessary to make sure you are getting enough sleep. In trying to fit in 15 or more hours of work each day, we tend to sacrifice our precious sleep. Lack of sleep, sleep disorders, and stress will dramatically reduce the quality of life.

LACK OF SLEEP

The average sleep duration is seven hours per night. The amount of sleep one needs is however individual. Even though we'd like to avoid sleeping every once in a while, we are not able to survive without sleep entirely. Severe physical and mental disturbances will occur, and eventually even death. While sleeping, we go through cycles of deep sleep, which alternate between periods of REM. These cycles repeat themselves around four to five times a night. But what really happens while we sleep?

A lot is going on while we sleep: our organs are regenerated, healing of wounds is accelerated, and memories are processed. And according to author Detlef Pape, sleep can also makes you thin. In his book *Schlank im Schlaf* (translation: "sleeping slim"— available only in German), the diet concept he mentions sets biorhythms and insulin levels in the center point. The pancreas releases the hormone insulin after eating so that blood sugar levels can be regulated. In his book, Pape explains that the body then absorbs the sugar molecules from the blood and stimulates the body to store fat instead of burning it for energy. In the long, up to five-hour breaks between meals, the pancreas is able to rest. The insulin levels will sink and the body will have enough time for the metabolic and digestive processes. The theory therefore states that by getting enough sleep and keeping levels of insulin secretion low, the body will not favor reserving fat during regenerating phases, and that sleeping can, in fact, make you thin.

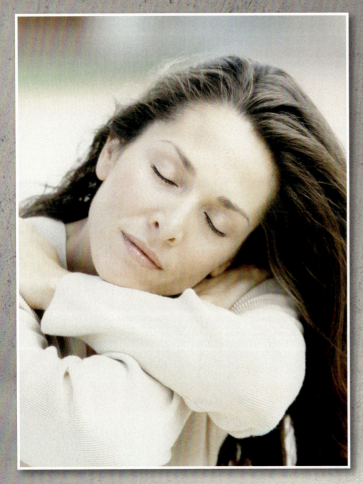

The body needs a certain number of hours of sleep to be able to recover. A good night's sleep is mentally and physically relaxing. If you chronically don't sleep well, you will be at risk of acquiring a poor functioning immune system, cardiovascular disease, stroke, high blood pressure, or suffer from obesity. A lack of sleep can also make you hungry. Studies have shown that insomniacs have higher levels of appetite stimulating ghrelin and leptin, the hormones that signal the body that it's had enough food. Leptin is produced in the fat cells. If too much leptin is produced, it apparently loses its effect. Because the values vary, it is assumed that people who don't get enough sleep can rapidly change from having no appetite to having cravings—cravings for unhealthy food.

If you suffer from constant fatigue, you most likely undergoing a painful struggle to get through the day. And if you come home from a hard day at work completely exhausted, there is little chance you'll have the energy to cook yourself something healthy for dinner. You'll most likely be tempted to reach for some junk food instead. Thus, a vicious cycle is born: in order for the body to optimally regenerate and stimulate the burning of fat, it needs enough sleep. If you don't get enough sleep, you'll have higher levels of the hormones ghrelin and leptin, which in turn will stimulate the appetite. Those who do not sleep enough have more cravings than those able to get in their required hours. And if you feel tired, you're not likely to find enough energy to make yourself something healthy and nutritious to eat.

CHAPTER 4

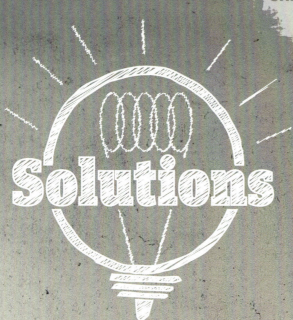

ELIMINATING BLOATING – QUICK FIX

In this chapter, we are going to show you how you can transform a bloated/fat belly into a nicely shaped slender belly. If you're only dealing with an unshaped belly due to bloating, then Chapter 1 is right for you. Give the 4-Day Quick Fix a try and you'll see how your belly and uncomfortable symptoms will improve.

Example: Saskia
Text from Saskia to Romy: "Hi Romy! Yes, of course you can use my photos. I unfortunately didn't take my weight and measure my waist. I didn't take the 4-Day Quick Fix seriously at first. Therefore, all I did was take a before and after photo."

"I am sooooooooo grateful to you for this plan. I've been in a constant battle with my bloating for the past few years and now, thanks to you, I know what is not good for me!!! I would be grateful for even more tips and recipe ideas. Can I buy a book from you? Kind regards, Saskia"

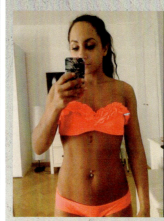 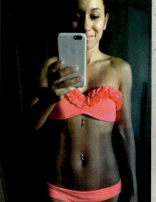

Before   *After*

FRUIT BELLY

If it's not only bloating that you're dealing with, but also fat deposits on your belly, you'll need longer than four days to address this. You'll find a lot of advice, strategies, and tips in this chapter.

> **IF YOU DO ALWAYS WHAT YOU DID, YOU WILL GET WHAT YOU ALWAYS GOT.**
> — Anthony Robbins

Your body is the result of your habits. If you're not happy with the way you are now, then you have to do something different in the future to change it.

I can hear you saying: "Yeah...but…" No, this is not the way it goes. Yes, this can make you feel uncomfortable. Yes, you have not done everything perfectly in the past. Yes, you are going to make some radical changes. Yes, it'll be tough and you'll experience many positive and negative experiences. Yes, you'll have to change some well-loved habits. Yes, you will be asked to change your old habits. And yes, you will be very pleased with your small and large improvements. And yes, others will be envious because you're successfully slim and happy!

This is life. We grow. We become stronger. And the best thing about Pure Food Paleo is that we become freer and no longer dominated by food.

LOSE WEIGHT – CHANGE YOUR LIFESTYLE

Theory: In order to lose body fat, there has to be a calorie deficit. Meaning, you have to eat less calories than you burn.

Practice: Change your lifestyle!

Please note! What does not work to change physically (at least not in the long run) is to eat less and exercise more.

The solution strategy to lose weight long-term, is not complicated. However, you've got to make the change in the right way. In short:

- Alleviate hunger
- Activate your fat metabolism
- Stay in fat metabolism phases longer
- More sleep
- Integrate fitness to activate/stimulate metabolism/hormones
- Have more fun and be more relaxed

Conclusion: Don't begin a limited time diet. Put the focus on changing your lifestyle, one that can be carried on until the end of life, that is healthy and enjoyable.

CHAPTER 4 | SOLUTIONS

You will be guided step by step through these six points. Beforehand, there's an important job for you to do. You'll need to take some time and a piece of paper or your diary and answer these questions honestly.

WHY DO I WANT A CHANGE?

What I wrote in my journal was:

- I want to have abdominal muscles that are visible
- I want to get rid of the bloating
- I want to get rid of the constipation
- I want to know what I can eat without causing digestive problems

I wanted it so bad that I didn't care what others thought about me or my plans. I wanted to reach my goal.

> JUST KEEP MOVING FORWARD AND DON'T GIVE A SHIT ABOUT WHAT ANYBODY THINKS. DO WHAT YOU HAVE TO DO, FOR YOU.
> — Johnny Depp

I was emotionally ready for a change.

BE EMOTIONALLY READY FOR A CHANGE

Why do I want to make a change to lose body fat?
It's most important to ask yourself the question—"why." What is motivating me to do so? What is the reason for making a change? And why is this reason so overpowering that I will stick to it and not fall back into my old bad habits?

The clearer you are, the easier it will be to stick with your plan and reach your goal. If the "why" is not coming from your heart, then you will always find excuses that will keep you from beginning or steer you off course.

Pressure from another person, family, or friend, is not reason enough to permanently change your lifestyle. If it's not coming from your heart, the good intention to change will be forgotten as soon as a crisis or stressful situation comes about.

Under certain circumstances, health risks can cause you to make a U-turn in life. A heart attack can turn a smoker one day into a non-smoker the next, because he doesn't want to continue risking his health. However there are other cases when a smoker has survived a heart attack (or cancer for that matter) and kept on smoking, as if nothing ever happened. I'm sure you're familiar with some of these cases personally.

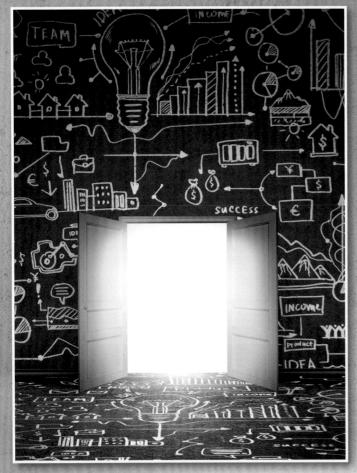

Personal aesthetic desires could be a strong inspiration. We want to look like the models on the cover of magazines and billboards. We see "perfect" figures and want to be like them, too. These people look completely different in reality—they too look like normal people. We strive for unreal Photoshopped perfection.

You must be aware that you can only minimally change your genetic body shape, such as your height and bone structure. What you are able to optimize are your muscle mass and body fat mass. Strong muscles aren't only the most important feature of health, they also shape our bodies. They tone and tighten the skin. Reducing your body fat levels to a healthy level—along with trained muscles—will bring out your individual, optimal, naturally perfect body.

It's important to know what you are able to change and what you cannot change. Accepting and appreciating yourself is an important factor to being happy. Be thankful for what you have been given. You can work on your attitude and lifestyle (diet, exercise, recreation, relaxation and social environment) in order to make improvements. A good plan and a positive attitude will support your intentions and bring you success. When your "why" is well defined and strong enough, the next step will follow. Where do you want to go, what kind of milestones will there be on the way and what must be done to get there.

LOSING BODY FAT – SETTING REALISTIC GOALS

First, we have to determine the starting position. There are different ways to do this: measure, weigh, and compare Before and After photos.

WEIGHT

You should weigh yourself at the same time of day in regular intervals. This will make it possible for you to keep track of your weight (trend line) without comparing yourself to other people.

IS WEIGHING YOURSELF DAILY NECESSARY AND/OR HELPFUL?

I've been weighing myself everyday since I was about 20 years old—for nearly 25 years now. Am I neurotic or maybe a bit of a control freak? I can deal with the number I see as I step on the scale and won't let it ruin my day. In the meantime, I now know the monthly, seasonal ups and downs, and fluctuations of my weight protocol. I know that during my menstrual cycle, I'm about three and a half pounds heavier (due to water retention). I know how much heavier I am the morning after "carb backloading" (restricting carbs during the day, conducting a depleting workout, and then aggressively refueling on carbs in the post-workout evening hours). I know from experience that in the summer, I tend to be at the top of my weight scale because

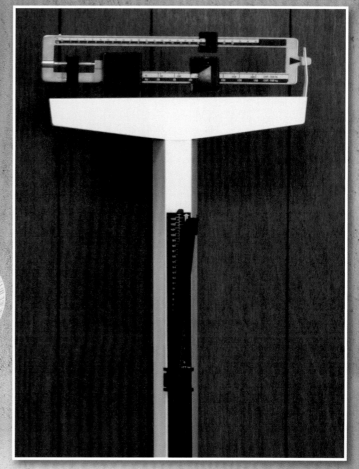

of water retention due to warmer temperatures. In the winter, when I tend to feel a bit cold, I tend to be on the lighter side. After flying, I need a good week before my weight adjusts itself, which is also due to inflight water retention. If I notice my weight keeps going up, and I haven't flown, or for no other apparent reason, then I become a bit more aware of my daily diet. I will sometimes leave out my evening snack or practice intermittent fasting (allowing my body to recover for long periods of time between meals—mostly between dinner and breakfast). Weighing myself is a part of my morning routine. It gives me information about my body—just as some take their temperature every morning (to determine the menstrual cycle) or measure their pulse (athletes).

If weighing yourself on a daily basis stresses you out because you don't see the desired number on the scale, then it's okay to weigh yourself less frequently. If seeing an undesirable scale reading leads to not eating all day to lose weight, only to then give in to cravings out of frustration, it's not worth it.

Weighing yourself daily –
University of Minnesota study
How the weight developed in a period of over two years in people who weighed themselves daily, weekly or never.

The results showed that the people who weighed themselves daily lost an average of 13 pounds. The people who weighed themselves weekly lost an average of 6 pounds. And the ones who never weighed themselves actually gained an average of 4 pounds.

The results of this study on weighing yourself daily supports the idea that it is beneficial to people who want to lose or maintain their weight. Weighing yourself daily can be an effective tactic, as it provides feedback on a regular basis. Even a small weight gain can be measured and controlled before it gets out of hand and, before you know it, have even more pounds on your belly and thighs.

It was also suggested that this method is not recommended for everyone. For people with eating disorders, stepping on the scale daily could possibly worsen unhealthy behavior.

BODY MASS INDEX (BMI)

Who doesn't know the BMI guideline from out of all the magazines and doctor visits?

Weight/height
If maintained within range then everything is okay.

WOMEN

Age	Range 1	Range 2	Range 3	Range 4	Range 5
18 to 24	<19	19 to 24	24 to 29	29 to 39	>39
25 to 34	<20	20 to 25	25 to 30	30 to 40	>40
35 to 44	<21	21 to 26	26 to 31	31 to 41	>41
45 to 54	<22	22 to 27	27 to 32	32 to 42	>42
55 to 64	<23	23 to 28	28 to 33	33 to 43	>43
65+	<24	24 to 29	29 to 34	34 to 44	>44

MEN

Range 1	Range 2	Range 3	Range 4	Range 5
<20	20 to 25	25 to 30	30 to 40	>40
<20	21 to 26	26 to 31	31 to 41	>41
<21	22 to 27	27 to 32	32 to 42	>42
<22	23 to 28	28 to 33	33 to 43	>43
<23	24 to 29	29 to 34	34 to 44	>44
<24	25 to 30	30 to 35	35 to 45	>45

1: UNDER WEIGHT   2: NORMAL WEIGHT   3: SLIGHTLY OVERWEIGHT   4: OVERWEIGHT   5: SIGNIFICANTLY OVERWEIGHT

Only this is not the whole truth. For example, for athletes with a very high proportion of muscles, these values are no longer valid. Or suppose you are at normal weight, but not physically active and have high levels of fat. Then are these values still correct?

Not really: While BMI provides a rough evaluation of whether our weight is within an acceptable range, it does not inform us of our risk of acquiring diabetes or cardiovascular disease. Not only the amount of fat should be considered, but also the distribution of fat. Those who have an "apple figure" (fat belly) are at greater risk than those with a "pear figure" (fat around the hips and thighs). In women, waist circumference should be below 31 inches and in men below 37 inches.

WHR (WAIST TO HIP RATIO)

To measure the waist to hip ratio, first the waist circumference is measured, then the hips. Then the waist measurement is divided by the hip measurement. For women, this value should be less than 0.85, and for men less than 1.0.

Which of these methods is better? Neither, if used on its own. It's better to use a combination of the two. BMI and fat distribution are the key factors.

DR. ALBERS –
HOW MUCH BODY FAT IS HEALTHY?

The WHO defines a body mass index (BMI) value of 25 to 30 as overweight; those with a value of over 30 are considered obese. It is easy to calculate your BMI since you only need your weight and your height. The BMI does not distinguish between high levels of fat and muscle mass—if the value is high, then you supposedly weigh "too much" for your height. Body fat percentage refers to the body fat percentage of total body weight. To calculate this is far more difficult, and in reality can never be 100 percent correctly measured. Hydrostatic (underwater) weighing, and the now more common DEXA method, are able to get more accurate values. When using the DEXA (dual-energy-x-ray absorptiometry) method, the body is scanned using x-rays (radiation dose is lower than used for TSA body imaging used at airports!). Conclusions on body fat, muscle, and bone mass are drawn based on the x-ray absorption. DEXA machines are quite expensive and are therefore available in only a few specialized centers. Because of this, it is more difficult for most of us to measure fat percentage values this way as compared to using the simple BMI. This is why no professionally accepted normal ranges of body fat percentages exist for men, women, or children.

Other body fat measuring techniques, including bioimpedance analysis (BIA) or skinfold measurement using a caliper, are much less accurate and depend heavily on the experience and qualifications of the person measuring. Not to mention that the results of the skinfold test are usually three or four percentage points lower than the more accurate DEXA measurement.

For these reasons, the following table is intended for use only as a guideline for the estimation of body fat percentage. It is based mainly on the experience of the authors and the few available data from studies.

DETERMINING BODY COMPOSITION BY MEASURING CIRCUMFERENCE

	VERY LOW HIGH PERFORMANCE TRAINING CONDITION	LOW GOOD TRAINING CONDITION	AVERAGE NORMAL RANGE	HIGH CAUSE FOR HEALTH CONCERN	VERY HIGH HIGH RISK HEALTH CONCERN
MEN	< 10 %	10–15 %	15–22 %	22–30 %	> 30 %
WOMEN	< 14 %	13–20 %	20–30 %	30–38 %	> 38 %

Women with very low levels of body fat (less than 12 percent) will often experience missed menstrual cycles, and in the long term will be at risk for bone loss (osteoporosis).

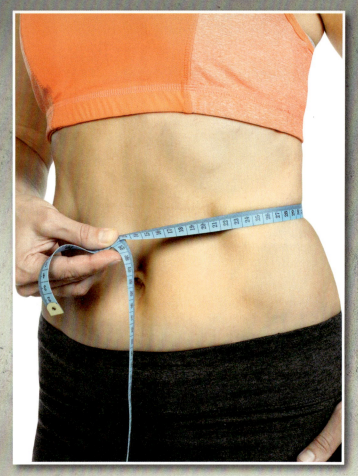

DETERMINING BODY COMPOSITION BY MEASURING CIRCUMFERENCE

You can do this with a flexible measuring tape, measuring different parts of your body (abdomen, waist, upper arms, thighs)—an important feature if you are training while losing body fat. Your weight could remain the same when you gain muscle mass and lose body fat simultaneously.

The shrinking measurements will clearly show that your body is changing in a positive way.

YOUR WAISTBAND: AN ALTERNATIVE WAY TO MEASURING YOUR CIRCUMFERENCE

Use a pair of pants as a reference. This is the way to go if the number on the scale stresses you out and ruins your day when you don't see the "right" number.

BLOOD TESTS

I recommend having your blood tested periodically. Blood tests do not show your change in weight, but they'll show you how your health has changed through dietary changes. It's better to discuss the results with a doctor who is familiar with reduced carbohydrate diets. It's important that the doctor can interpret the results correctly, and not give you outdated nutritional advice.

WHAT IS A REALISTIC GOAL?

Once you have the base data, you can define your goals. Let's say you weigh 165 pounds and have a fat percentage of 30 percent (48.5 pounds body fat), and you'd like to reduce your body fat percentage 10 percent.

A defined goal should be as precise and specific as possible. The abbreviation SMART will help you determine an effective goal.

S = specific ->		Reduction of body fat (not just body weight)
M = measureable ->		10 percent less body fat/ 20 percent of body fat percentage
A = accepted ->		Yes, I want to lose weight in a healthy way and not experience the yo-yo effect. I will introduce new habits
R = realistic ->		Yes, I have 10 weeks until my wedding day, and I'd like to look slim and happy in my wedding photos.
T = time ->		Until my wedding day, April 15, 2015 (today is February 1, 2015)

DO WE REALLY NEED A GOAL?

Without goals, actions are unthinkable. They enforce you to act on your commitment, based on your knowledge and intentions, to achieve your goal. As soon as you've defined your "SMART" goal, and when you feel comfortable and can identify with it, the next step is your personal plan and strategy.

STRATEGICALLY CHANGE YOUR LIFESTYLE

INFORM YOURSELF FIRST AND GAIN KNOWLEDGE

Knowing what, when, and how I need something is crucial. To know how something functions (for example how body fat is biodegraded in the body) is helpful, but not absolutely necessary to reach your goal. I don't want to know, for example, exactly how my TV works. I just need to know how to turn it on, how to change the channels, and to adjust the volume.

CREATE AN OPTIMAL STARTING POINT

Examples:
- Reorganize the kitchen
- Give or throw away all industrially processed foods
- Think about what kind of exercise/sport plan you'd like to do and buy any necessary equipment
- Create a meal plan
- Choose recipes and print them out
- Write a grocery list
- Go shopping
- Precook for the upcoming week

REORGANIZE PROCEDURES
- Think through your daily routine/write it down
- Prepare your breakfast the night before
- Google restaurants ahead of time and check the menu out
- Go for a 30 to 60 min walk (slip it in your daily routine)
- Schedule time in the evenings to cook
- Etc.

INFORM OTHERS

There are two strategies here. The offensive strategy: I will let everyone know about my goal and ask for support. Or the secretive strategy: you don't tell anyone or just a few trusted people and begin introducing new habits without attracting attention. For example, not eating any more bread or pasta. You don't need to explain your actions while continuing to cook as usual for the rest of the family.

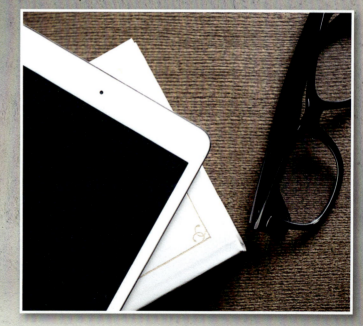

Avoid trying to convince others to join you. It's better to play the part of a pioneer and surprise everyone with your positive improvements. Who doesn't want to be slimmer, healthier, and happier? When everyone notices the positive changes, this will be the perfect time to tell everyone your story and what you did to make it possible. Maybe then, your partner may want to join you. With kids it's a bit different—just slowly introduce more and more healthy food and simply don't buy any more junk food. They will get used to eating healthy food with time. Pressuring them into eating differently could have the opposite effect and will very rarely bring success. Patience and endurance are a lot more effective.

CHANGE YOUR PLAN

> DO IT BADLY, DO IT SLOWLY, DO IT FEARFULLY, DO IT ANY WAY YOU HAVE TO, BUT DO IT.
> — Steve Chandler

Don't wait too long and overthink it. Just do it! Sometimes you'll make better decisions than other times, and there may be times when you fall back into your old habits or "slip-up." This is normal. We didn't learn to write mistake-free over night, did we? And once we did learn how to write, we still make mistakes every once in a while—through carelessness, time pressure, or pure ignorance. I'll say it again: This is completely normal. Be prepared for "slip-ups" and learn from them. This is why the next step is so important.

DEFINE EMERGENCY SITUATIONS

It's important after a slip-up to get back on course and not write off the rest of the day and continue slipping-up. Making a wrong decision is not putting your goal in danger. You have learned from your mistake—the next time you're in the same situation, you'll make a better choice and decide differently.

> LET YOUR PAST MAKE YOU BETTER, NOT BITTER.
> — Author Jackie

CELEBRATE MILESTONES

Separate large goals into stages. It's good for your soul to celebrate each completed stage. This motivates you to keep on going. When you are having a hard time, you can look back on your achievements. This will give you strength and lift you up in low times.

KEEP GOING

Endurance and persistence will lead you to success. By remaining focused and acquiring good habits, you will remain successful.

> WE ARE WHAT WE REPEATEDLY DO. EXCELLENCE, THEN, IS NOT AN ACT, BUT A HABIT.
> — Aristotle

PURE FOOD PALEO PRINCIPLES

1. PRINCIPLE: NATURAL FOOD
We eat natural food. The major criterion for the selection of natural food is that the food we eat can also be raw. What can we eat raw? Vegetables, fruit, meat, fish, eggs, nuts, seeds, water, and raw milk. We avoid everything that we cannot eat raw: grains, potatoes, legumes, etc.

We are not naturally raw food eaters, although Pure Foods in raw form are well tolerated. Many foods when cooked are more easily digested, taste better, and its nutrients are better absorbed. Cooking our food makes our diet more interesting.

2. PRINCIPLE: UNPROCESSED FOOD
We buy unprocessed food with no artificial additives, such as flavorings, plasticizers, stabilizers, thickeners or dyes. All artificial additives hinder our natural satiety (feeling full). A good example is artificial sugar. It has zero calories, but will stimulate the appetite and cause the body to feel hungry. This is why it is used to fatten animals in the meat industry.

3. PRINCIPLE: LOCAL FOOD
We eat locally grown food whenever possible. Transporting distances are shorter and we put less of a burden on the environment. We buy our food directly from the farmer or producer with appropriately reared animals and organically grown fruits and vegetables.

4. PRINCIPLE: SEASONAL FOOD
Local seasonally grown fruit and vegetables have the advantage that they can be harvested ripe. They have more flavor and are more nutrient dense. Mostly, seasonal products are cheaper than imported products from distant lands.

5. PRINCIPLE: ORGANIC FOOD
Organic food does not necessarily contain more nutrients. There is no consistent evidence to prove this in scientific studies. However, it is true that fewer pesticides are used, protecting the benefits of the food's natural state by lessening exposure to toxins.

In the case of animal products, the organic label means that the animals are treated appropriately and humanely (access to outdoors, fresh air, and sunshine) and fed organically. This is very important to me—first of all because of the wellbeing of the animals, and secondly because organic meat, fish, and eggs contain more natural nutrients (for example omega-3, vitamin K).

We can only get and stay healthy by eating healthy food. Animals that are treated with antibiotics and fattened with grains and artificial sugar are not a healthy source of nutrients.

6. PRINCIPLE: BALANCED MACRONUTRIENTS

Pure Food Paleo is a balanced diet. Macronutrients are evenly divided into about 30 percent protein, 30 percent carbohydrates, and 40 percent fat in order to maintain your weight. If it is your goal to lose body fat, the amount of carbohydrates is temporarily reduced and replaced with healthy fat.

In this type of diet, we pay a lot of attention to healthy, natural fat. Natural fat does not make us fat. It's the starchy carbohydrates that stimulate our fat reserves to grow.

A Pure Food Paleo Diet focuses on the following natural healthy fats found in: meat, fish, poultry, and eggs (of course from healthy/happy animals), avocado, coconut oil, clarified butter, butter, ghee, nuts, and small amounts of extra virgin olive oil. Apart from the nuts and olive oil, all of these fats contain little or no omega-6, which is pro-inflammatory.

Avoid all industrially produced vegetable oils, such as sunflower oil, peanut oil, soybean oil, etc. These oils are highly processed and have the tendency to become rancid very quickly. They also contain high amounts of omega-6 fatty acid, which can cause our omega-3:omega-6 ratio of 1:2 to become off balance. If omega-6 fatty acids get out of hand, this will trigger inflammation in the body.

7. PRINCIPLE: GLUTEN

We eat gluten free. Gluten is a sticky protein found in grain and is difficult to digest. It is often not completely broken down into single amino acids. This leaves undigested particles behind. These protein particles are called peptides. Depending on the condition of the intestinal mucosa, they can pass through the mucosa (leaky gut syndrome) and enter the bloodstream. Gluten peptides can also trigger allergic reactions, causing swelling and inflammation. In contrast to an insect bite on your arm where the swelling is easily identifiable and noticeable, you normally don't notice the swelling triggered by an allergic reaction in your intestines.

Even more difficult to detect is allergic inflammation in the brain. You do not notice the swelling of brain tissue as you do with your skin—itchy, soreness, swelling. Allergic inflammation in your brain—such as a reaction to gluten peptides—is very subtle, often felt as a "foggy feeling" in your head.

Grain does not contain any essential nutrients and can therefore be eliminated from your diet problem free.

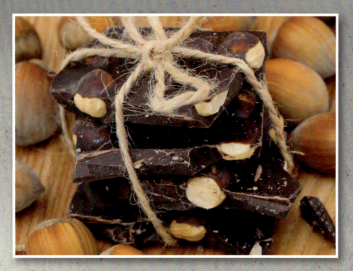

8. PRINCIPLE: SUGAR

Our sugar intake is reduced to the minimum. And by sugar, we aren't just talking about table sugar. We are talking about all types of sugar—honey, fruit sugar (fructose), maple syrup, and all artificial sugar. The less sugar we eat, the more sensitive our taste buds become. Our sweet tooth will automatically disappear and we will appreciate the taste of natural sugar.

Artificial sugar is not an alternative. It is not good for you and will confuse your body's inner intelligence. Our brain will continue to want more sweet stuff and will not be satisfied with nutrient-rich, natural food. We won't feel satiated and satisfied. Sugar is an addictive substance, similar to alcohol, heroin, and other drugs.

If you're in the mood for something sweet, it's better to reach for some good quality chocolate with no artificial additives and at least 72 percent cacao content. Or have some fruit or a homemade dessert made with small amounts of sugar. It is important that you consciously eat and enjoy it as a special treat.

9. PRINCIPLE: DAIRY PRODUCTS

Dairy products are unfortunately so "damaged" through pasteurization and homogenization that the human body is no longer able to properly digest them.

On the other hand, raw milk, in its natural state, directly from the udder, is better tolerated by most people.

There are several reasons why raw milk is better tolerated. The enzymes in the milk are not destroyed with high heat (pasteurization) and actively support the human digestive process.

Due to the homogenization process, the two milk components—water and cream—are combined so that the cream doesn't settle on top. The disadvantage of this nice, consistent, homogenized milk is that your digestive system does not rec-

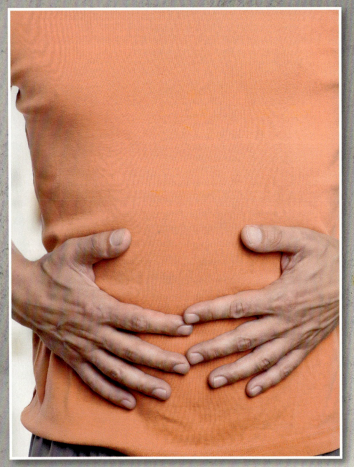

ognize these newly combined fat-water units. They are foreign, not digestible, and can trigger gas, diarrhea, stomach cramps, constipation, chronic intestinal inflammation, and other problems.

It's important to mention here that not everyone has the ability to digest even raw milk and its products (raw milk butter, raw milk cheese, etc.) due to a deficiency of lactase (digestive enzyme in the stomach) or casein (milk protein) intolerance.

In order to find out if you may be lactose intolerant, it's best to eliminate all dairy products from your diet for at least one week and observe how you feel. It's also possible to have a blood test, but this test is less reliable.

10. PRINCIPLE: LEGUMES

We avoid legumes because they are difficult to digest. The composition of macronutrients (fat, protein, and carbohydrates) is not optimal. Legumes contain not much protein but a lot of carbohydrates and anti-nutrients (lectins and saponins), which make the intestinal walls porous (leaky gut syndrome), triggering chronic inflammation in the body.

DRINKS

THIRST—WATER

To satisfy your thirst, drink water. Drink pure water from the tap, if you're lucky enough to have clean, drinkable water in your home. Otherwise, drink still (non-carbonated) bottled water, preferably in a glass bottle.

If you find plain water boring, you can "spice it up" with a squeeze of lemon juice or add some peppermint leaves. You could also make a pot of herbal tea (without sugar)—fruit tea is not recommended since it is mostly artificially flavored. Let the tea cool and drink it throughout the day.

Mornings, you can drink coffee or tea with breakfast, or drink a butter coffee instead of eating breakfast. Don't use tea/coffee to quench your thirst, and don't drink it with milk and sugar. Coffee is a stimulant and should be not drunk in large doses. Tea (black, white, or green) contains antioxidants, which can relieve infections and strengthen your immune system. What's important when drinking coffee and tea is to make sure you drink good quality products. Roobios tea is a great caffeine-free alternative, which also contains valuable antioxidants.

ALCOHOL—IN MODERATION

Alcohol is a toxin. The body does everything it can as quickly as possible to eliminate a poison from its system. Alcohol is immediately metabolized in the liver, and the liver won't stop working until the alcohol is completely eliminated from the body. Consequently, alcohol disrupts the digestion, prevents the absorption of nutrients, and can trigger inflammation in the digestive organs.

As long as the body is busy with eliminating the alcohol, fat and body fat reserves will not be broken down. There have been studies showing the health promoting factors of alcohol. You can do your own research on the Internet, and I won't deny it. However, while red wine contains certain health promoting ingredients, alcohol is still a poison. And, how your body reacts in order to eliminate it remains reason enough to be critical.

If you'd like to make an exception, then stick to good quality, gluten free products, such as one or two glasses of red wine or a shot of rum (made of sugar cane), brandy or cognac (made of grapes), or a good quality tequila (made of agave). I didn't mention beer, since it's better to avoid it. Beer contains a lot of gluten and carbohydrates, which in turn will promote a nice, round, beer belly.

> To satisfy your thirst, drink water. Drink pure water from the tap, if you're lucky enough to have clean, drinkable water in your home. Otherwise, drink still (non-carbonated) bottled water, preferably in a glass bottle.

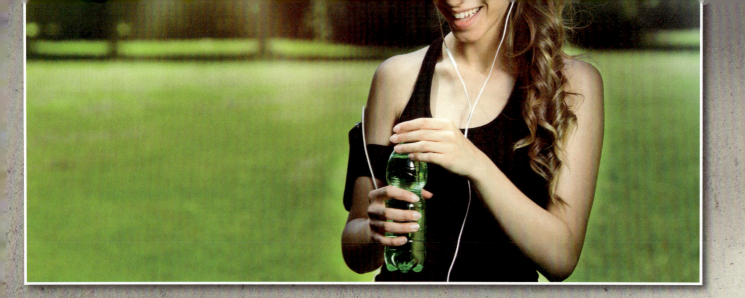

FINALLY
These recommendations do not have to be 100 percent strictly followed. The longer you follow Pure Food Paleo, the easier and more normal each day, weekends, invitations, parties, and holidays will be.

It's important to be strict with foods that make you sick by eating even the slightest amount. This is the case with celiac disease, where the smallest amounts of gluten can cause severe problems.

With children, it's better to make dietary changes fun to avoid a prolonged state of stress. At home, eat Pure Food Paleo. Offer a large selection of different kinds of vegetables and fruit, so that your kids can choose for themselves what kind of healthy food they'd like to eat. This way, there will be less of a battle and you'll all be able to eat a relaxing meal that's better digested.

Whenever possible, kids should take part in shopping, too. If they are able to choose healthy food they enjoy, they will be more likely to eat it.

Adults have to make the right choices while shopping. Look closely at the labels of so-called "kids products." Very often, they are full of unexpected ingredients such as sugar, fructose, flavorings, dyes, etc. It's the parent's responsibility that these kinds of food are not available at home. If the refrigerator and cupboards are full of junk food, it's no wonder that the kids will want it, having become addicted to it from an early age.

Eating out or on the go with kids is a bit more of a challenge. The wide range of (high-sugar) tempting products is outrageous. Children very often don't understand why they are supposed to resist the temptation. They don't understand that eating unhealthy food has a negative impact on how they feel. We parents, on the other hand, do—hyperactivity, allergies, eczema, poor concentration, and runny noses are just a few of the many symptoms that are triggered by eating unhealthy food.

Children need natural food that tastes good and provides the essential nutrients needed to be healthy, happy, and intelligent kids.

TESTIMONIAL

"G" AND HIS BELLY—9 POUNDS LESS BODY FAT IN 25 DAYS—CONGRATULATIONS!!

"G"'s parents are Italian and his mama spoiled him from an early age with Italian delicacies. In his youth, he was able to burn the carbohydrates from all the pasta, bread, and desserts he ate without getting fat. In his early 40's, "G" noticed that it wasn't as easy anymore to maintain his ideal weight. Despite regular exercise, his belly kept on growing. When he was not able to exercise for a while due to an accident, his belly grew even bigger and rounder. He tried to eat less, but even this didn't help. On the contrary, this just slowed down his metabolism and caused even more problems to arise—sleep disorders, high blood pressure, and chronic pain.

"G" did the 4-Day Quick Fix first and then continued for four more weeks with Pure Food Paleo Low Carb, following the recipes and meal plans in the book. As recommended, he kept a food/feelings diary and came by on a regular basis to weigh in, measure, and to photograph his belly.

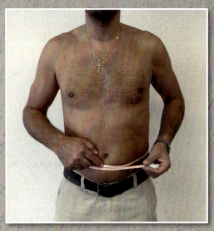

Starting point
November 4, 2014
Weight 209 lbs
Body fat 29.2%
Muscle mass 148 lbs

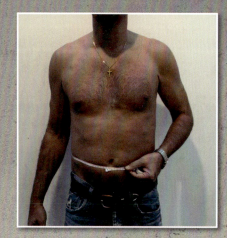

After the 4-Day Quick Fix
November 8, 2014
Weight 203 lbs
Body fat 28.9%
Muscle mass 145 lbs

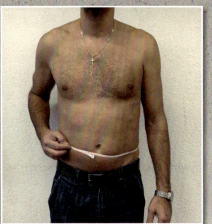

After two weeks of Pure Food Paleo Low Carb
November 23, 2014
Weight 200 lbs
Body fat 27.8%
Muscle mass 144 lbs

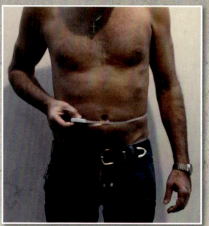

After three weeks of Pure Food Paleo Low Carb
November 29, 2014
Weight 200 lbs
Body fat 26.1%
Muscle mass 147 lbs

WHAT DO THESE NUMBERS MEAN?

These numbers show nicely how "G" didn't just lose weight, but that most of the weight lost was body fat. His muscle mass remained fairly constant at 148 pounds. He lost a total of 9 pounds and 3.1 percent body fat.

It's interesting to hear how he felt and what changes he noticed during the four weeks.

- The recipes were easy to follow and tasted good
- I was satisfied with the portions. The first few days, I experienced an uncomfortable feeling of being "too full" but after a few days, this went away.

Romy: Changing your diet is always a challenge for your body to adjust to. But it's a good sign that you recognize and notice the changes.

Romy: If the bloated ("too full") feeling does not go away after a few days, you should check if there could be an intolerance to one of the foods on the Quick Fix diet plan.

- It is time consuming to cook the meals. I have to make it more of a daily routine.

Romy: Planning and organizing is important so that you can successfully change your lifestyle.

Romy: With time, you'll get used to this and planning the meals, shopping lists—cooking will become a part of daily life.

- **During the Quick Fix, I became somewhat impatient and almost a bit aggressive. I believe I felt this way during times when I normally would calm myself down with carbohydrates (bread, sugar).**

Romy: This is a typical sign of addiction. Our brain is dependent and requires carbohydrates (sugar). In moments like these, when the brain releases a strong feeling of desire, it can be extremely difficult emotionally. With "G", he took out his aggressions on himself and others.

Romy: It's important in situations like this to be aware of what is happening. As soon as the emotional challenge is addressed, the disproportional intensity will fade. Over time, the brain will realize that if nothing happens after sending out these signals (no sugar), it will learn not to long for it anymore.

Romy: It's also important during this difficult phase to explain to family and friends why you are acting this way—exaggerating or overreacting. Clearly communicate that it has nothing to do with them, but purely mental and physical withdrawal symptoms.

Romy: By addressing the challenge and communicating with others, it will be easier to deny temptation. You've figured it out yourself. The withdrawal symptoms are not to be underestimated, not in their frequency or severity. It is especially easy to lose control in emotionally difficult situations, which could cause you to reach for that bar of chocolate.

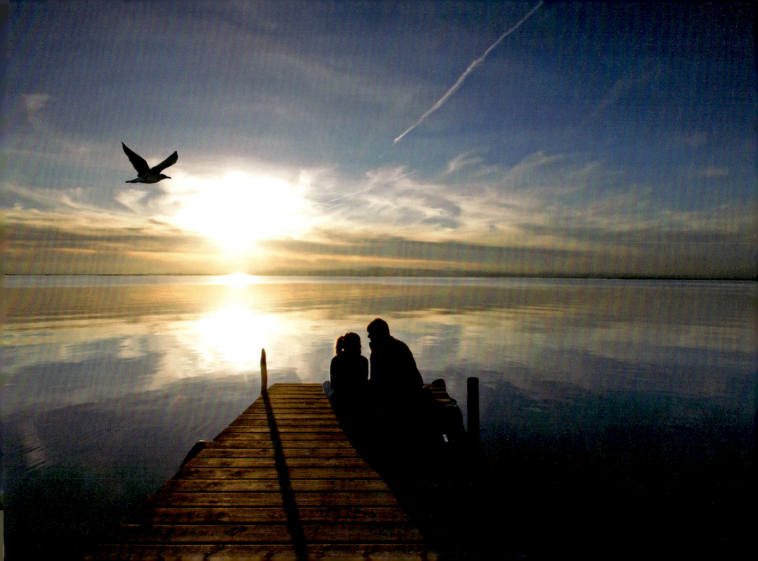

- Not eating anything between meals was difficult for me at first—not because I was hungry, simply because of my habit to grab something out of the fruit bowl or the chocolate "stash."
  Romy: Habits are not to be underestimated. They function automatically in our brain. You'll need a strategy in order to avoid going back to your old ways.

- It took a few weeks to adjust, but now I don't crave carbohydrates anymore.
  Romy: We all have habits in life, but we are able to change each and every one of them.

- During the day, I often feel tired and worn out.
  Romy: It's difficult for "G"'s body to adjust to using fat and fat reserves as energy sources. It's taking a lot of energy just for the adjustment, which can cause fatigue and lack of energy. This is a good sign, even though it's not very pleasant while adjusting.
  Romy: Once the body is acclimated to using fat and body fat for energy, it will be much easier. The day will come when "G" gets up in the morning and thinks: Wow! What happened to me? I feel like I could climb the highest mountain!

- My strength training performance has somewhat declined.
  Romy: Despite his fatigue, "G" went for daily 30 to 60 minute walks. He didn't, however, force himself to incorporate strength training sessions. It's important to listen to your body, in this case. Once the energy has returned, he can train more intensively.

- I now sleep longer and deeper, feeling more refreshed in the mornings. This improvement in my sleep alone has made the diet worthwhile. I want this to continue in the future.
  Romy: This is very common when people switch to eating a Paleo diet. Everything seems easier when you're able to get a good night's sleep and allow your body to rejuvenate and recover during the night. It is a part of the positive spiral that automatically occurs through a Paleo lifestyle.

- I felt hungry for the first time in years. It was a feeling that felt foreign to me. During the Quick Fix, I became aware of it. Not because I was forced to starve myself—the portions were very generous and more than satisfying—but because I tended not to eat too much at mealtimes and avoided eating snacks in between. I now like the feeling of being hungry; it gives me a sign that my body is properly functioning and is able to send the right signals at the right time. It also really increases the pleasure of eating.
  Romy: Paleo allows us not only to live more consciously, but once all the artificial substances and toxins are eliminated from our body, we are able to really "feel" ourselves. Our body will let us know exactly what and how much natural food it needs.

What are "G"'s plans for the upcoming weeks? He wants to continue this new way of eating and to keep on reducing his body fat percentage until his six-pack becomes visible.

"G" lost 9 pounds of body fat in just 25 days. He walked 30 to 60 minutes a day and did some light strength training every once in a while. To further boost his body to burn fat, he could incorporate HIIT into his training schedule.

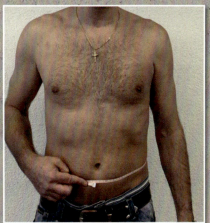

After three months
February 13, 2015
Weight 195 lbs
Body fat 24.8 %,
Muscle mass 146 lbs

> *Official dietary guidelines*
>
> Respective to the history and development of dietary recommendations up until 1950, the focus was on the prevention of malnutrition. This is especially true in Europe during World Wars I and II. During this time, diabetes and obesity were not the focus of attention. Only since the second half of the last century have dietary guidelines considered a connection between diet and the health risks of diet-related diseases. The main organizations responsible: in Switzerland (SGE), in Germany (DGE) and in Austria (ÖGE). Now, most western counties have a national nutritional organization, which implements current dietary guidelines to encourage improvements in public health. Besides the reference values for an average adult person, there are specific recommendations issued for children, pregnant women, seniors, athletes, and other population groups beyond the standard recommendations.
>
> The Swiss Associations support new studies that favor low carbohydrate intake and higher fat intake. Excessive fructose intake is officially classified as a health hazard, according to the Swiss. This encourages the balanced nutrient ratio of Pure Food. The international organization WHO has also released nutrient and vitamin recommendations according to regional and cultural differences. For example, the recommendations in Asia contain none or very little dairy products, whereas in Europe, this is not the case.
>
> In summary, the international trend is to steer away from large amounts of carbohydrates and favor more high quality fat. Also, consuming large amounts of fructose is questioned more and more, particularly added sugars and juice. The macronutrient ratio of Pure Food corresponds exactly to the current knowledge and has been proven most effective in recent studies.

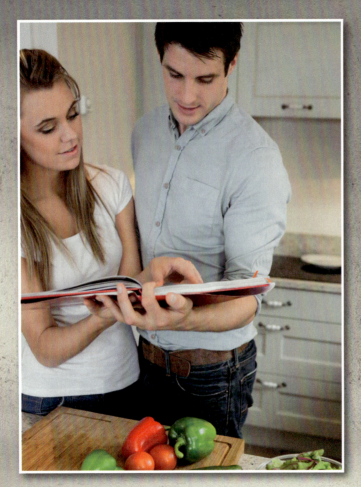

LOSE BODY FAT – IMPLEMENT YOUR PLAN

You can implement your plan step-by-step or pick out individual points. You'll have the greatest success if you can add another point every week, and in six weeks integrate all six points into your life.

ALLEVIATE HUNGER
- Use meal plans and recipes
- Apply Pure Food Paleo principles
- Eat when you are physically hungry
- Keep a food/feelings diary

ACTIVATE YOUR FAT METABOLISM
- Reduce carbohydrates
- During two to three weeks, gradually eat less carbohydrates to more easily make the change and to reduce fatigue

REMAIN IN FAT METABOLIZING PHASES LONGER
- Avoid eating starchy carbohydrates in the mornings (bread, cereal, etc.); use the breakfast recipes
- Eat dinner early in the evening and avoid eating any snacks before going to bed
- Make the break between dinner and breakfast as long as possible

SLEEP MORE
- Regular restful sleep makes you more relaxed
- You feel more balanced and make better decisions
- Your hormones are more regulated and assist in reducing body fat
- You are more resistant to stress

INTEGRATE FITNESS TO ACTIVATE/STIMULATE YOUR METABOLISM/HORMONES
- Do two to three HIIT per week
- Stretch on a regular basis
- For beginners, first learn the HIIT techniques and exercises with a trainer so that you learn how to do them correctly

HAVE MORE FUN AND BE MORE RELAXED
- Plan "me time"
- Play and be lazy
- Meditate
- Spend time with friends and family

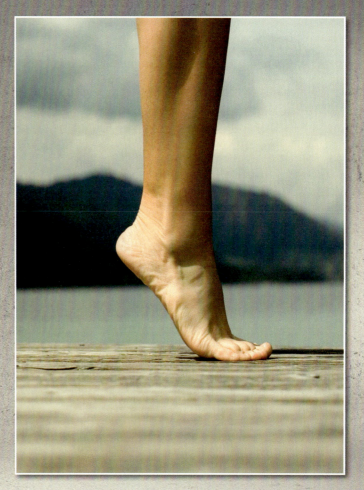

CHAPTER 4 | SOLUTIONS

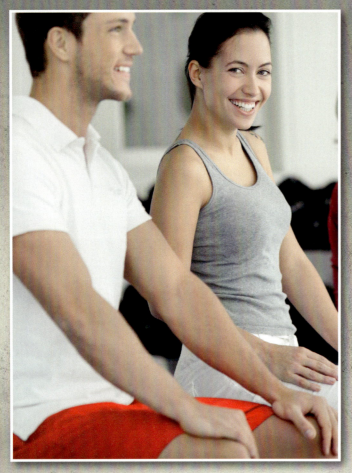

> **No Yo-Yo Effect with Pure Food Paleo Diet**
> Because you never have to go hungry with Pure Food Paleo, and you receive all of the necessary nutrients, your body isn't afraid that it's not getting enough nutrients. Your body has no need to increase its fat reserves. On the contrary, your body will tap into its fat reserves to provide great amounts of energy when necessary.
>
> And when is this necessary? When all the carbohydrate reserves are empty and you don't fill them again by eating more carbohydrates.
>
> However, this wonderful natural process will only work smoothly and without any side effects if you have "trained" your fat metabolism. You can do this by eating a carbohydrate reduced diet (Pure Food Paleo), making sure there are long breaks without snacks between meals, getting enough rest and relaxation (balanced hormones), and practicing short intense fitness sessions (HIIT).

OPTIMAL BODY (BELLY) POSTURE

Look at these pictures then go look at yourself in the mirror. And? Which picture can you relate more to: the picture on the right or on the left?

A flat stomach has a lot to do with having good posture, either while standing or sitting. With a slouched back, hanging shoulders, a sunken in chest, you're only contributing to your big belly. The extreme opposite—chest stuck out, the neck relaxed and jaw pulled back into the throat, arched pelvic or knock-knees—belong to the characteristics of poor posture. Poor posture will

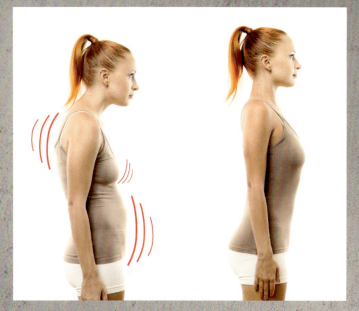

INSTRUCTIONS FOR OPTIMAL BODY (BELLY) POSTURE WHILE STANDING

- The plumb line is centered from the top of the body to the bottom
- Head, shoulders, pelvis, hips, knees, and feet are straight
- Shoulders are square yet relaxed
- Pelvis and head are erect
- Spine is elongated and the neck is extended
- Thighs are slightly rotated outwards
- Knees face forward
- Feet are v-shaped

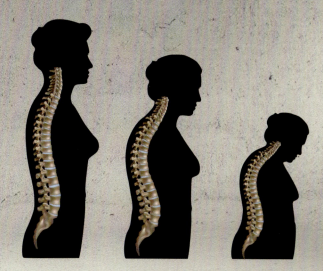

not only affect the way you look, but can also be the cause of many health problems: backache, neck and shoulder problems, pain in the knees and hips, headaches, sleep disorders, circulatory disorders, pinched nerves/sensibility disorder, hallux valgus (crooked toes), arthritis, etc. As you can see, the list is very long. It is important to pay attention to your posture, to protect your back and the rest of your body too. Do it for the sake of looking good and for your health.

CHAPTER 4 | SOLUTIONS

Unfortunately it has become habit for us to sit incorrectly hours on end. The human anatomy is meant for movement. Besides regular and frequent exercise, it's important to also practice correct posture while sitting.

INSTRUCTIONS FOR OPTIMAL BODY (BELLY) POSTURE WHILE SITTING

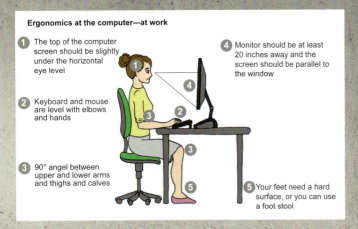

Even when you sit down, you should make sure your spine is erect. This will make it easier for you to sit upright and also avoid developing thoracic curvature by slightly tilting your pelvis forward. The muscles and intervertebral disks will be evenly strained, the abdominal area relaxed, circulation in the legs is improved, and breathing is free. If you begin to slouch your back during the day, stabilize your posture with the backrest.

Try to avoid getting stiff by changing your sitting position throughout the day. Sometimes lean a bit forward, then lean a bit back and maybe sit upright for a while. Making even small movements are good for your muscles and spine. Distribute your weight sometimes more to the right and then to the left, slide back and forth on your chair or tilt your pelvis forward and back again.

Did you know that you automatically relax your shoulders when you rest your arms on the armrests? And, that muscle tension in your neck and shoulders can be reduced by putting the palms of your hands on the keyboard? Give it a try!

FITNESS ROUTINE: HIIT – HIGH INTENSITY INTERVAL TRAINING

WHAT TYPE OF TRAINING IS MOST EFFECTIVE WHEN IT COMES TO BURNING FAT?

There is a lot of misleading information out there on what is the best way to train to burn fat. Such as always training on the same machines, in the same tempo, for the same amount of time for every session.. Your body gets used to these exercises quickly and needs some new stimuli. The same goes with the intensity of the workouts.. Working out for an hour on the cross-trainer at the same level (aerobic training/pulse at 110 to 130) will not bring you closer to your goal. Interval training (HIIT) or Tabata training methods have been proven to be a more effective approach. You will definitely be more challenged, but your workouts will have a long-lasting effect (known as the afterburn effect).

HIIT is a short yet performance demanding training system that consists of interplay between intense strenuous phases and active recovery periods.

There are different ways to train HIIT using various training plans—depending on the duration and actual intensity of the intervals.

For example, an intense, strenuous phase could be sprinting, and the recovery period could be walking. Meaning that an interval consists of a strenuous activity and a break. The interplay between the two will promote the burning of body fat, which has been proven in many scientific studies. Just a few weeks of training this way can result in a noticeable reduction of abdominal fat.

Extent of HIIT Training

HIIT workouts take anywhere from 20 to 30 minutes. Three sessions a week is all it takes and you will already notice the improvements. Compared to 30 to 60 minutes of aerobics, you will burn twice the amount of fat in a shorter amount of time. In addition, your basal metabolic rate will increase, resulting in more energy (calories) burned while resting. HIIT also has an effect on various hormones. This would include the growth hormones that are responsible for building muscle.

Which HIIT methods are connected to each other?

In order to burn fat, two of the most effective methods are connected: high intensity training and interval training.

Training with high intensity will challenge your maximum performance. The more active your muscles are, the more oxygen will be needed. Endurance athletes will aim for the highest possible oxygen intake. The more oxygen your body can process per minute while training, the higher the performance. Training to the near point of exhaustion will lead to an "afterburning effect" lasting up to 48 hours after the workout. Fat will be burned even in the recovery phase.

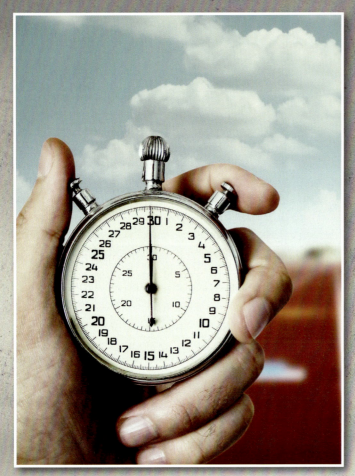

Interval training alternates phases of higher and lower intensity. The objective of interval training is to boost the metabolism, which is achieved at a much higher rate than when working out at a constant, steady pace. The body burns a lot more calories in a 20-minute HIIT workout than in a 20-minute workout at a constant intensity.

TABATA

In addition to the HIIT training method, there is also Tabata. Tabata training (metabolic training) was developed by Izumi Tabata at the National Institute of Fitness and Sports in Tokyo. In his study, he found that just five four-minute workouts a week over a period of six weeks produced maximal oxygen consumption and improved anaerobic capacity. The shorter the workout, the higher the levels of intensity should be. A typical interval lasts 20 seconds, followed by a pause of 10 seconds. As a rule, eight intervals are carried out (total time: four minutes). In endurance training for example, sprint for 20 seconds then walk for 10 seconds. In strength training, do as many reps as you can for 20 seconds, then rest for 10 seconds before performing the next exercise as fast as you can. The difference between HIIT and Tabata is the duration and intensity of intervals. As a general guideline, the shorter the training duration, the higher the range of intensity and the longer the breaks.

DR. ALBERS – STRENGTH TRAINING AND WEIGHT LOSS

Losing weight requires a negative energy balance—or expending more energy than we take in over time. This can be achieved by regular endurance training (aerobic). However, the necessary training period is much longer than we might expect it to be. It would take a woman at least 15 hours of intense jogging at 6 miles/hour before achieving energy consumption that corresponds to 2 lbs of fat tissue. Strength training requires less energy per time unit than intense endurance, but indirectly shows greater effects on body composition.

By applying only endurance training while restricting calorie intake, 70 to 80 percent of the weight loss will consist of fat—however 20 to 30 percent of the weight lost will be muscle mass. This not only leads to loss of muscle tissue, but will also slow down metabolic activity—or decrease resting metabolic rate (RMR) since muscle will burn fat (energy) even while resting. This will increase the possibility of the yo-yo effect if endurance training is used for the sole purpose of weight loss. Intensive strength training, on the other hand, can preserve muscle mass even if there is a calorie deficit—and will reset the metabolism to burn rather than save, which tends to happen with endurance training. Effective strength training will have an effect on energy consumption 24 to 48 hours after training. Intense endurance training, to the point of exhaustion, will affect post-training energy consumption by burning an estimated 50 calories, whereas intensive whole-body strength training will stimulate the metabolism to burn 200 to 600 calories within the following 48 hours. Even beginners are able to stimulate the resting metabolic rate (RMR) and burn up to 600 calories in the recovery period after strenuous strength training. That's equivalent to a whole bar of chocolate! This process is called "afterburning."

The increased afterburning effect that occurs after strength training compensates for the low energy consumption during the actual training, as compared to endurance training where more energy is consumed while training but there is less of an afterburning effect. With strength training, you may not notice a reduction in weight, but you will notice an increase in muscle mass and a reduction of stubborn fat mass. Strength training is optimal for toning the body, reducing subcutaneous fat, and allowing the well-trained muscles to be visible.

PRIORITIZE RELAXATION

GET ENOUGH SLEEP

The average person will spend one third of his or her life sleeping. Is sleeping a waste of time? Not really. In order to balance out relaxation and stress, you'll need to get enough sleep. Sleep is essential for the body and mind. Circulation, breath and pulse are all slowed down while sleeping. The brain, however, continues to work at peak performance: it processes the events of the day. Sleep is viewed by most people as something natural and necessary. Sleep only becomes an issue when it's disturbed. Those who can't sleep well understand how important sleep is for our body and mind.

Since the invention of the light bulb, we no longer sleep according to the natural daily rhythm. We prolong our days until late in the night and spend hours watching TV or sitting in front of the computer—even though it's way past our bedtime. Simply put, we are stealing time from our sleep. We can't determine our sleep patterns alone, because our inner clock is ticking and provides the rhythm. Individual sleep needs differ. It's best to experiment and find out how many hours of sleep you need in order to feel refreshed and full of energy. Take notes and make comparisons. If you have enough energy during the day to properly function and perform, then you're probably well-rested. Feeling a bit low on energy at midday, however, is completely normal.

SLEEP—A NEW TREND

Because we are sleeping less and less, there has been an increased interest in the subject of sleep. According to a study, our resting rhythm has become disturbed due to smart phones and other devices. Being reachable 24/7 is making us a sleepless society. Therefore, the topic of sleep is becoming more and more popular. A survey done recently showed the following theories on sleep:

Sleeping is a lifestyle
- We invest in our beds, mattresses, even sleeping "gadgets."

Sleeping as a status symbol
- Those who sleep well are more ambitious, creative, and successful

Power-napping
- Power-napping is now encouraged. Having a power-nap after lunch can give you strength and power for the rest of the day.

Sleeping becomes public
- Sleeping pods at airports, sleeping masks, and nap pillows make it easier to sleep in public

Lack of sleep
- Sleep has also become a topic in preventative health care. Fatigue eventually can lead to heart problems, high blood pressure, etc.

Sleep as a key factor of success
- If you sleep enough and sleep well, you'll be empowered—not only in professional sports, but also in society

SLEEP PATTERNS
Studies confirm that children who do not have a regular sleep schedule suffer in mental development. But, what about adults? What happens when we go to bed at 3:00am on the weekends and at 10:00pm on the weeknights? Irregular sleep patterns like this are similar to those working night shifts. With time, irregular sleep patterns can negatively effect your health. By the way, catching up on sleep on the weekends does not work. Just because it's the weekend and you don't have to get up, doesn't mean you should just stay in bed longer. You should get up as soon as you are awake. Your body appreciates routine.

SLEEP AND DAILY LIFE
Sleep is the source of relaxation and recovery. Not getting enough increases your risk of getting mentally and physically sick. Sleep disorders can cause inflammation in your body leading to atherosclerosis (the building up of plaque inside the arteries). Headaches, high blood pressure, and gastrointestinal problems could all be the result of not getting enough sleep. While you sleep, the events of the day are processed to support the learning function. Our immune system works at full speed while we sleep. Not enough sleep reduces the activity of antibodies. Have you ever wondered why you can sleep eight hours without food? The answer is the hormone leptin. This appetite suppressing hormone is distributed while you sleep. Chronic sleep deprivation can disrupt the balance between leptin and ghrelin (appetite stimulating hormones).

GOOD SLEEPING CONDITIONS
There are different stages of sleep that last a period of about one to two hours: light sleep, stable sleep, deep sleep, and REM (rapid eye movement). During deep sleep stages, the body regenerates and builds important building blocks for organ reparation. Your brain operates at a slower rate and the amount of stress hormones released is very low. We dream during the REM stage, while the brain is active, similar to the waking state. Mental recovery takes place during the dream stage. On average, people sleep six to eight hours a night. The optimal amount of sleep depends on the quality of sleep. If you are able to get your six to eight hours of sleep without any disruptions, you will feel rested and refreshed in the morning. How is the quality of your sleep at the moment? Do you feel relaxed and rested when you wake up in the morning? How many hours of sleep do you need in order to feel well

and to master your daily life? Maybe these tips will motivate you to give it some thought and make any necessary changes.

TEMPERATURE

Open your windows in the morning and before going to bed at night to get some fresh air in your bedroom. The room temperature should be at around 64° F and humidity should be at about 50 percent. Your bedroom should be fairly dark, especially if you're a light sleeper. Electronic devices can disturb you—put your radio and TV on stand-by mode. Make sure that there are no electronic devices that illuminate the room.

BEDROOM VERSUS OFFICE

Your bedroom is not an office. Therefore avoid leaving documents such as bills and invoices lying around that could cause you to worry and could keep you up thinking in the middle of the night. Solve your problems before you go to bed. If this isn't possible, make a list of things you need to do and worry about it tomorrow. Your bedroom should be tidy and you should feel comfortable and safe. Grey and green tones tend to be relaxing.

RITUALS

Find out what makes you feel good and what calms you down before going to bed—make yourself a cup of tea (soothing and calming herbal teas), a relaxing bath, quiet music, or going for an evening stroll. Maybe read a few pages of your favorite book. Or

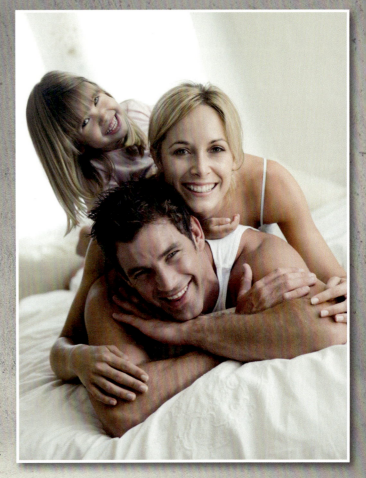

FRUIT BELLY

you could start meditating and set a ritual of meditating before going to bed every night. Meditating quiets the mind—which is perfect for going to sleep. Avoid caffeinated beverages, having a full stomach, or drinking too much alcohol—which may help you fall asleep easier but will affect the quality of sleep. Also try to avoid unnecessary adrenaline kicks—don't do any sports right before going to bed.

PEACE
High-noise levels can cause stress. But not everyone can choose where they live.. Not everyone has the luxury of living in a quiet place in the country. There are ways to block out sound and light—good blackout curtains and earplugs.

DIET
Before going to bed, the process of digestion should be completed. You should eat dinner no less than three hours before going to bed. It's wise to avoid caffeine at least six hours before bedtime. Alcohol impairs sleep quality and contributes to a light, superficial sleep.

DR. ALBERS – LACK OF SLEEP AND OBESITY

Sleeping less than six hours a night can, after a few days/nights, result in adverse hormonal changes. This could lead to an increase of the hormone cortisol, a typical stress hormone. This could cause a reduction of muscle mass, especially in the extremities. Chronic increased cortisol levels will also encourage redistribution of fat mass to the middle of the body, creating the beginning of a fat belly. This increase of visceral fat tissue has long-term negative effects on the metabolism and blood vessels (increased risk of diabetes, heart attack, and stroke). In addition, high cortisol levels caused by a lack of sleep lead to poorer glycemic regulation, so that carbohydrate-rich foods cause blood sugar and insulin fluctuations, which in turn leads to cravings and obesity. Appetite behavior and satiety regulation are affected even after a few nights of less than six hours of sleep. The brain sends false hunger/satiety signals to the body triggering sweet and fatty cravings, which in turn will contribute to excess calories and weight gain.

Chronic lack of sleep will cause loss of muscle mass, increased fat tissue, increased abdominal circumference, and poorer appetite regulation. These factors prove that in the long run, chronic lack of sleep indirectly promotes the development of diabetes mellitus.

REDUCE STRESS

It's important that you have a healthy attitude towards stress. Stress cannot be completely eliminated from your life. You encounter stress factors that you are not even aware of (Vester, Frederic, 1978: Phenomenon Stress). And many factors simply cannot be avoided, such as noise.

The symptoms vary from person to person. Everyone was born with certain physical weak points that stress especially will reveal. It may affect your stomach, while someone else may get headaches and yet someone else will have heart problems.

RECOGNIZE STRESS

Mostly it's the high demands on yourself that trigger stress reactions. How would it be if you changed the way you think? If you keep thinking the same way, you tend to get caught in a loop. Constantly asking yourself "What should I do?" or worrying for hours about something will only increase your feelings of stress and fear. Bad feelings can become even stronger so that the body and mind are not able to recover (chronic stress). As soon as you get some distance from what is bothering you and are able to look at the situation from a different perspective, you will be able to escape the worrying process. Many people find it helpful if they write down their thoughts, feelings, and solution suggestions.

DODGE STRESS

Very often you have no influence on stress factors. You can, however, determine how you deal with stress and how you react. A good example is the weather and work-related demands. You can become upset about the rainy weather and complain about all the work that you have to do, turning your mood into a bad one. Or, you can accept that it's raining and bring an umbrella with you and make the best of the day. And the same goes for your job. You can put yourself under an enormous amount of pressure, constantly tell yourself that you have so much to do and so little time. But, you're only mentally planning a future full of worries and fear. Another possibility is to make a "to do" list and complete tasks one job at a time. Think positively and look at everything you've already accomplished, not only what you haven't accomplished. Talking positively to yourself is particularly important for successful stress management and avoiding stress all together. This way you automatically feel better and have higher potentiality for success.

EXERCISE MORE

Exercise—walking, jogging, tennis, bike riding, yoga, strength training, etc.—promotes relaxation. Consistent, steady, rhythmic movements, deep breathing, and physical exertion will relax you. Exercise also makes you tired, content, and happy. At the same time, we are able to mentally relax while we exercise. Worries are suddenly forgotten as we hike up the mountain in the fresh air. You clear your head and are able to relax.

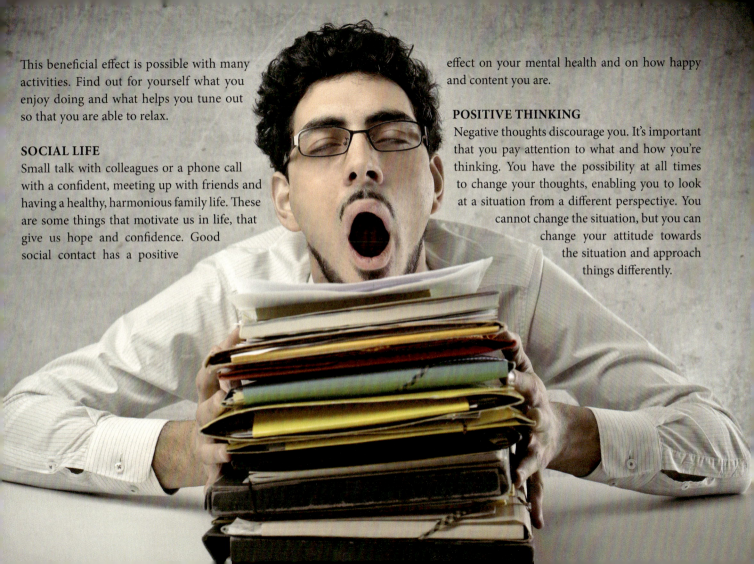

This beneficial effect is possible with many activities. Find out for yourself what you enjoy doing and what helps you tune out so that you are able to relax.

SOCIAL LIFE
Small talk with colleagues or a phone call with a confident, meeting up with friends and having a healthy, harmonious family life. These are some things that motivate us in life, that give us hope and confidence. Good social contact has a positive effect on your mental health and on how happy and content you are.

POSITIVE THINKING
Negative thoughts discourage you. It's important that you pay attention to what and how you're thinking. You have the possibility at all times to change your thoughts, enabling you to look at a situation from a different perspective. You cannot change the situation, but you can change your attitude towards the situation and approach things differently.

PUT YOURSELF ON THE TOP OF THE LIST

Do you make yourself happy? Do you do what's good for you? If you neglect yourself because of all the stress, you need to do something about it. Schedule time for yourself and consciously enjoy that time. How your "me time" looks is up to you. What do you enjoy doing? It could be a nice warm bubble bath after a hard day at work, or a pedicure, a massage, or going to the opera. A bike ride with a good friend or maybe enjoying a day alone without the family. It's best to write your "me time" in your calendar and take it seriously.

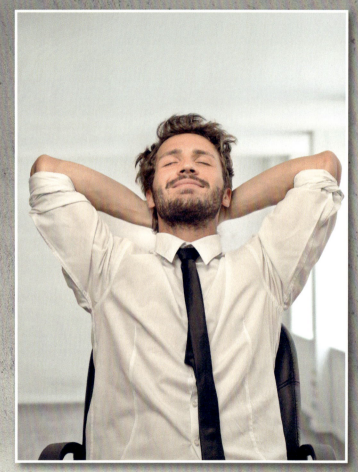

EMOTIONS

> **IT IS NOT THE THINGS THAT BOTHER US, BUT OUR INTERPRETATION OF THEIR SIGNIFICANCE**
>
> Epictetus

EMOTIONAL PERCEPTION

The feelings historian, Ute Frevert from the Max Planck Institute for Human Development, is of the opinion that we are taught emotions, not born with them. We can basically say that emotions first have to be recognized and understood. This may sound quite logical, but the ability to recognize, to correctly interpret and to make the appropriate decision on which emotion to have, is far from easy. We are not given this ability, we have to learn it. How many times a day are we angry or sad and we don't know the reason why we feel this way? To interpret and classify our feelings is not always easy and takes practice.

The ability to perceive your own emotions, the feelings of others, and to interpret them correctly can be measured with an emotional intelligence test (EQ). In contrast to the IQ test, mathematical and verbal skills are not tested. If a person is unable to perceive emotions correctly, he/she could mostly likely be suffering from alexithymia—an inability to read emotions.

ADDRESSING EMOTIONS

We are not meant to only be happy in life. We all go through rougher and darker moments, and this is normal. Personal life crises tend to shape our personality more intensively than carefree stages in life. In order to not allow crises to turn into a complete disaster, we must learn to deal with them. But it's not always easy to make the right decisions. Our habits tend to get in the way and make life even more difficult. How can I manage to turn defeat and frustration into something positive? Deepak Chopra and Rudolf E. Tanzi give the following advice in the book *Super Brain*:

Should I solve this problem, come to terms with it. or completely forget about it?

Who can I turn to for advice on finding a good solution for this kind of problem?

How am I able to look inside myself for the solution to this problem?

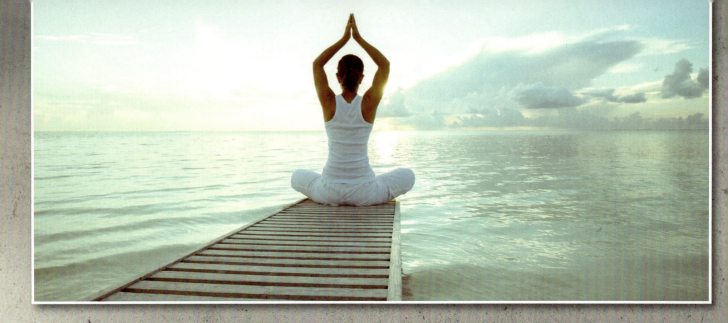

COME TO TERMS WITH EMOTIONS AND ACCEPT THEM
There are several ways to come to terms with emotions and to accept them better. A very good way is meditation. Meditating makes you more confident, attentive, and focused. It allows you to become even more aware of your surroundings and yourself. Meditation focuses on being alert and allows you to cope with stress and anxiety in a more productive way.

Meditation works with the mind. It's about becoming aware of who you are and how you function. The whole day, our thoughts circle around in our brains. When we meditate, we put these thoughts to rest and your mind concentrates on your breathing. It takes patience to learn how to meditate. At the beginning, it can be helpful to attend or participate in a meditation class. You could also try it on your own—sitting upright, Indian style, your eyes lowered but open, the palms of your hands placed face down on your thighs, focused on your breathing. If thoughts begin to drift in, then put the focus on your breath again. Try doing this for 10 minutes, 20 minutes, or longer.

HOW TO KEEP A FEELINGS DIARY

Write from your soul. Writing can help you become more aware of your emotions, and will help you to interpret and understand them better. In a diary, you'll find the most intimate thoughts and desires, and writing is often used as a form of therapy. The most well known diary ever is that of Anne Frank. Instead of drowning herself in her feelings, she put them down in words.

Expressive writing stimulates the cognitive process. The complex process of emotional experiences are reviewed and structured in memory.

By expressing emotions and practicing self-control while writing, you support a healthy way of dealing with negative emotions. Try your expressive writing in the following way:

- Go to a place where you feel comfortable. It doesn't matter what time it is; it doesn't have to be necessarily right before going to bed.

- Write about something that emotionally touches you, something that's important to you. The topic can vary daily, although it may be better to stick with the same topic for a few days.

- Write for 15 minutes for at least three or four days. It's possible that on the third or forth day, you may have difficulty writing more on the topic. But this has a positive effect in the end.

- Be honest with yourself and what you write. Remember, paper can always be burned.

- You may feel a bit sad after you've finished writing. This will fade within a few hours. If you feel as if it's stirring up too much, then you do not have to continue with the exercise.

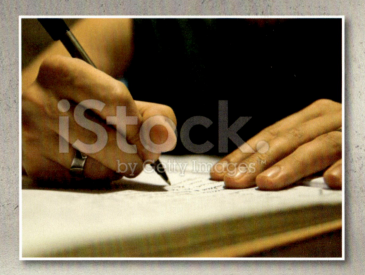

CHAPTER 4 | SOLUTIONS

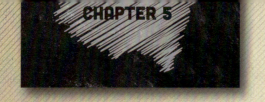

CHAPTER 5

Planning MEALS

FRUIT BELLY

MEAL PLAN INFORMATION

MEAL PLAN 1: PURE FOOD PALEO LOW CARB

Pure Food Paleo Low Carb is designed so that the carbohydrate content is greatly reduced to promote the burning of body fat.

There is no reason to go hungry. If the portions specified in the recipes don't make you satiated (full), then feel free to make more and eat until you've had enough. (But don't overeat!)

> As soon as your body has become accustomed to using fat and fat reserves for energy, you will feel less hungry. By eating nutrient dense food, your body will be satisfied and the breaks between meals will become longer without you even noticing it. Many feel, for the first time ever, free of cravings.

MEAL PLAN 2: PURE FOOD PALEO

Pure Food Paleo is less restrictive and allows gluten-free carbohydrates in moderation. This plan is perfect for those who would like to stabilize and/or maintain their weight. During the week, lunches are designed (marked in blue, pgs. 124-125) so that you can select/order them in a restaurant or cafeteria. If you cook lunch and dinner at home, you'll find more recipes in Chapter 6.

If you eat out at a restaurant in the evenings, you may choose a meal similar to one of the lunch meals. With Meal Plan 2, you could go to a Japanese restaurant and order mixed sashimi. Rice is naturally gluten free, so you may have a small portion of rice with your sashimi. Make sure you ask for gluten free soy sauce (tamari). Every Japanese restaurant has it nowadays.

If you don't care for one of the recipes in the meal plan, you may substitute it with another one. You may also eat the same meal more than once a week if you'd like.

The meal plans are designed so that you can get a feel for the individual ingredients and proportion sizes of a meal.

Tip: Cook a double recipe and eat half the next day, or freeze it for another day. This will reduce the time you spend in the kitchen.

MEAL PLAN ONE
PURE FOOD PALEO LOW CARB

WEIGHT LOSS

	BREAKFAST	SNACK (OPTIONAL)	LUNCH (AT A RESTAURANT)	DINNER	DESSERT (OPTIONAL)
DAY 1	Apple/Coconut Muffin	Butter Coffee	Beef/veal cutlet (no sauce or gravy) with vegetables (no potatoes!)	Cold Avocado/Cucumber Soup with Feta	Paleo Bounties
DAY 2	Butter Coffee	1 oz beef jerky or prosciutto ham	Fish filet (sautéed in butter or olive oil) with vegetables	Pumpkin Soup with Chicken Breast	Coffee Ice Cream
DAY 3	Butter Coffee	Butter Coffee	Grilled chicken (¼) with vegetables	Fish Package with Beet Salad	Berry Soup
DAY 4	Frittata	1 oz olives	Beef tartare or gluten free burger (without the bun) with vegetables	Thai Soup	Macadamia Nut Cookies
DAY 5	Smoothie	1 oz raw milk aged cheese	Tuna salad with vegetables	Zoodles with Shrimp	1 oz raw milk aged cheese
DAY 6	Breakfast Burger	3-1/2 oz. cucumber	Salad with sliced meat/chicken	Sashimi Puzzle	Chocolate Mousse
DAY 7	Coconut Berry Crunch Muesli	Butter Coffee	Sunny side up eggs with bacon and sautéed tomatoes	Spinach Topped with Salmon	Paleo Bounties

DAY 6 & 7: WEEKEND!

FRUIT BELLY

MEAL PLAN TWO: PURE FOOD PALEO

WEIGHT MAINTENANCE

	BREAKFAST	SNACK (OPTIONAL)	LUNCH (AT A RESTAURANT)	DINNER	DESSERT (OPTIONAL)
DAY 1	Butter Coffee	Butter Coffee	Grilled chicken (¼) with vegetables	Cauliflower Steak with Poached Eggs	Paleo Bounties
DAY 2	Coconut Berry Crunch Muesli	1 oz beef jerky or prosciutto ham	Vegetable salad with tuna	Ground Beef and Tomato Stew	Coffee Ice Cream
DAY 3	Breakfast Wrap	1 oz olives	Steak with vegetables	Thai Soup	Chocolate Mousse
DAY 4	Smoothie	20 plain Macadamia nuts	Vegetable salad with eggs	Cauliflower Steak with Poached Eggs	Apple Topped with Crumble
DAY 5	Blueberry Muffin	Butter Coffee	Fish filet with vegetables	Cauliflower Steak with Poached Eggs	Macadamia Nut Cookies
DAY 6	Smoothie	1 oz raw milk aged cheese	Pumpkin Soup with Chicken Breast	Sashimi/sushi with seaweed salad	Berry Soup
DAY 7	Breakfast Burger	Butter Coffee	Cold Avocado/Cucumber Soup with Feta	Paleo Burger with Sweet Potato Fries	Banana Crunch

DAY 6 & 7: WEEKEND!

CHAPTER 5 | PLANNING MEALS

CHAPTER 6

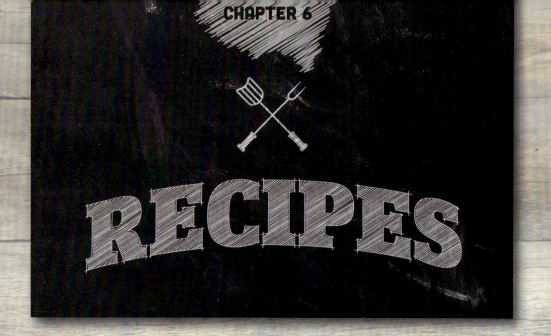

RECIPES

RECIPE INFORMATION

I have put together some recipes for you that are delicious and tasty. They are easy to cook and are made of food that you can easily get at the local grocery store or farmer's market. In some cases, the ingredients will be available at the health food store.

You can eat any recipe at any meal. For example, the breakfast options can also be eaten at lunch or dinner, with the exception of butter coffee (caffeine), which should only be drunk before lunchtime. Caffeine can affect your sleep, even if you don't seem to have difficulties falling asleep.

Organic food is preferred, which is less contaminated with pesticides, toxins, and drugs (antibiotics, etc.).

More specifically, I'd advise you to only purchase meat and animal products from humanely reared and fed animals, primarily for the benefit and health of the animals. But also because the fatty acid composition is modified in the meat of conventionally reared and artificially fattened animals. The amount of omega-6 becomes unnaturally high and can cause inflammation in our body. In addition, animals that are not humanely raised are sick more often and are treated with high doses of antibiotics. The remains of these toxic drugs accumulate in the fat of the animals.

Yes, organic food is more expensive than conventional food. If you buy seasonal produce directly from an organic farm or farmer's market, you can minimize costs. Organic products are said to contain more nutrients, so you will be satiated with smaller portions and more mentally and physically satisfied.

There are a few products that you cannot find at the grocery store or supermarket. Information on where you can find some of these products is on pg. 205.

The recipes are inspirations. I hope that you will try them out according to your own taste, using seasonal, local, and natural food—and that they inspire you to experiment and improve them to your liking.

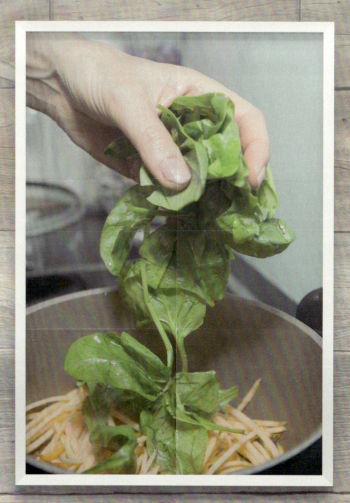

CHAPTER 6 | RECIPES – GENERAL INFORMATION

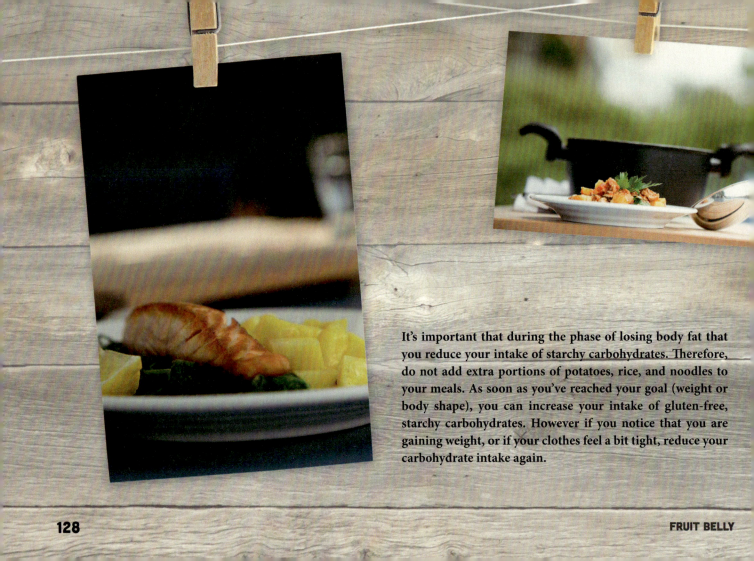

It's important that during the phase of losing body fat that you reduce your intake of starchy carbohydrates. Therefore, do not add extra portions of potatoes, rice, and noodles to your meals. As soon as you've reached your goal (weight or body shape), you can increase your intake of gluten-free, starchy carbohydrates. However if you notice that you are gaining weight, or if your clothes feel a bit tight, reduce your carbohydrate intake again.

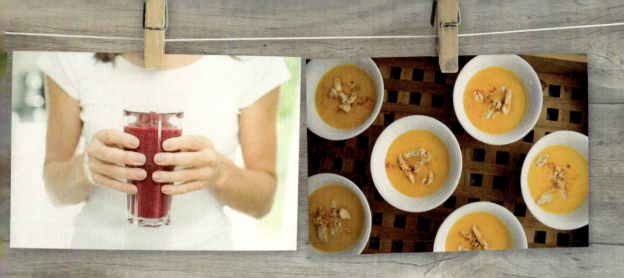

You are not allowed to be hungry and count calories! Eat as much of the meals as you'd like until you feel comfortably satiated. But do not eat more just because you want more! If you feel hungry between meals, first try drinking a big glass of water and wait 20 minutes. If you still feel hungry, eat a Paleo snack.

Keep snack portions to a minimum! Wait at least 20 minutes and drink a glass of water before reaching for another snack.

The desserts are here to show you that even with a reduced carbohydrate diet, small treats are allowed. You can enjoy one dessert a day, eaten directly after either lunch or dinner. The desserts included contain low amounts of carbohydrates compared to traditional desserts.
Desserts are optional.

CHAPTER 6 | RECIPES – GENERAL INFORMATION

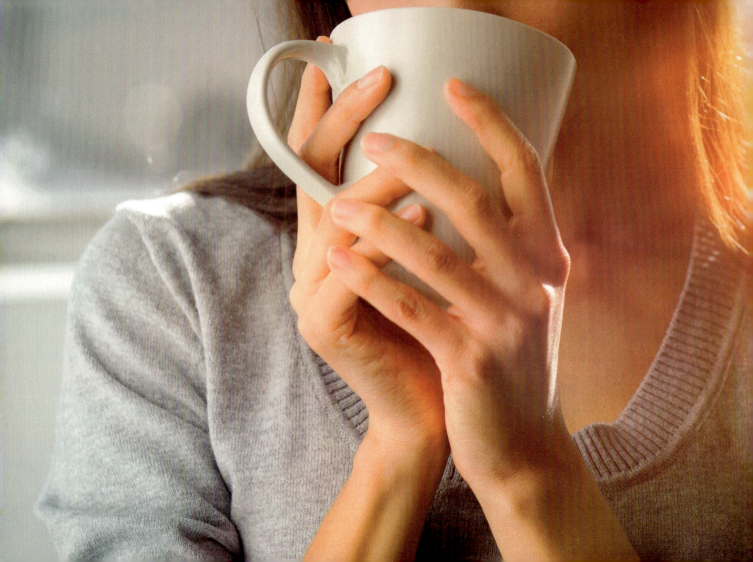

Breakfast

Breakfast is the most important meal of the day. What we eat for breakfast will determine whether our body will turn to its fat reserves or will adapt to burning carbohydrates for energy throughout the day. It doesn't matter if your breakfast is big or small, or whether it is in solid or liquid form. What's important is what it consists of.

Eating starchy carbohydrates for breakfast will put a stop to fat metabolism, and will trigger the body to turn to carbohydrates for a quick energy source for the remainder of the day.

RECIPES - BREAKFAST

APPLE AND COCONUT MUFFINS

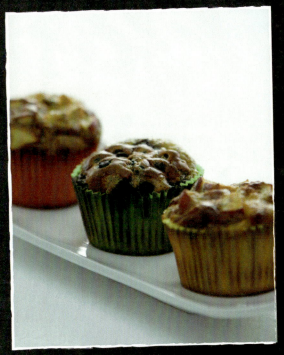

PREPARATION TIME: 40 MINUTES

INGREDIENTS FOR 8 MUFFINS:

- 8 eggs
- 3 oz coconut milk (containing only water and coconut)
- 2 oz honey liquid
- 2 oz desiccated coconut (health food store)
- 2 oz instant gelatin or vanilla protein powder
- 1 tsp vanilla extract or powder
- 1 tsp ground cinnamon (optional)
- ½ pound fresh apples
- 2 tsp baking powder

Preparation:
1. Preheat the oven to 350° F. Prepare muffin pan with paper cups.
2. Wash and dry the apples, remove the core and cut into small pieces. Mix all ingredients, except the apple, with a hand mixer or in a food processor until a smooth batter forms.
3. Carefully fold the apple pieces into the batter and pour the mixture into the paper cups prepared in the muffin pan. Bake for 30 to 35 minutes.

BLUEBERRY COCONUT MUFFINS

Same ingredients as in the Apple and Coconut Muffins recipe, except that the apples are replaced by ½ pound (fresh or frozen) blueberries.

IT IS EVEN QUICKER IF THE DICED VEGETABLES ARE PRE-COOKED IN THE MICROWAVE.

- 5 eggs
- 8 oz cooked ham or cooked chicken breast
- 8 oz zucchini
- ¼ lb tomatoes
- 8 oz carrots
- 1 Tbs clarified butter (ghee)
- Fresh herbs (such as chives, parsley, basil)
- Sea salt and black pepper
- Freshly grated parmesan cheese (optional)

Preparation:

1. Preheat the oven to 350° F. Line a small baking pan with parchment paper.
2. Wash and dice the vegetables into equal-sized cubes. Melt the clarified butter in a skillet and lightly sauté the diced vegetables. Spread the vegetables on the prepared baking pan.
3. Cut ham or chicken breast into cubes and place on top of the diced vegetables.
4. Rinse, dry, and chop the herbs. Briskly whisk the eggs in a bowl. Add the herbs and season with salt and pepper.
5. Pour the egg mixture carefully over the vegetables and meat cubes and bake in the oven for about 30 minutes. Once the egg mixture is golden brown and firm, take it out of the oven.
6. If desired, sprinkle with parmesan cheese. Can be served warm or cold.

RECIPES—BREAKFAST

FRITTATA

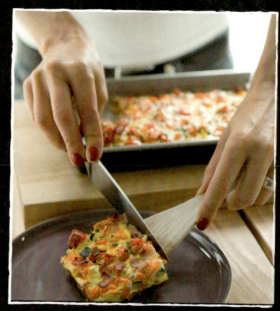

 PREPARATION TIME: 15 MINUTES

 INGREDIENTS FOR 2 TO 3 SERVINGS:

 THE FRITTATA CAN BE STORED FOR UP TO 4 DAYS IN THE REFRIGERATOR. IT IS AN IDEAL TAKE-AWAY BREAKFAST.

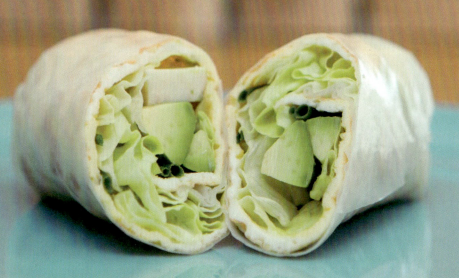

Breakfast Wrap

PREPARATION TIME: 15 MINUTES   INGREDIENTS FOR 2 SERVINGS

- 4 pieces of rice paper/spring roll wrappers (large)
- 4 eggs
- 3 oz raw milk cheese (parmesan or pecorino)
- ½ avocado
- 4 lettuce leaves
- salt
- black pepper or cayenne pepper (very spicy)
- tamari (gluten-free soy sauce)

ALTERNATIVE: SUBSTITUTE THE CHEESE WITH COOKED HAM

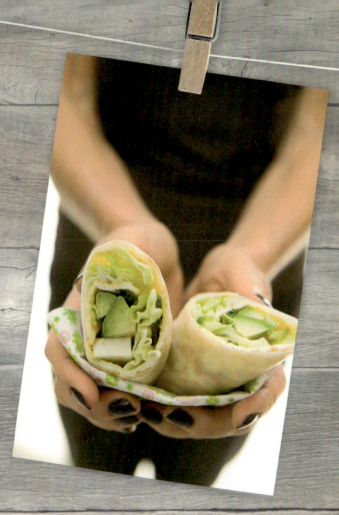

Preparation:
Soak the rice paper wrappers one at a time, according to the instructions on the package.

1. Finely grate the cheese or slice into thin strips.
2. Whisk the eggs in a bowl and season with salt and pepper or 1 teaspoon tamari.
3. Cut avocado in half, remove the pit and take off the peel.
4. Thinly slice.
5. Using a small non-stick frying pan, make small (about 6 inch) omelettes. Set aside.
6. Lay the pre-soaked rice paper on a damp cloth.
7. Place a small omelette in the middle of the rice paper. Add lettuce, avocado and cheese.
8. Now tightly, but carefully, roll the rice paper half way, then fold in the two sides and continue rolling until the wrap is completely rolled.
9. Eat immediately or wrap in cellophane for an ideal take-away breakfast.

RECIPES – BREAKFAST

COCONUT BERRY CRUNCH MUESLI

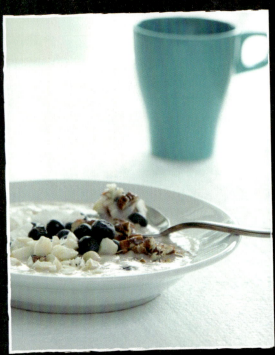

PREPARATION TIME: 10 MINS

INGREDIENTS FOR 1 SERVING:

- ½ banana
- ¼ cup coconut milk
- ¼ cup water
- 1-½ Tbs protein powder or instant gelatin
- 5 whole unsalted macadamia nuts
- 10 unsalted pecans halves
- 1 Tbs coconut flakes
- ¼ lb blueberries (fresh or thawed)

Preparation:
1. Purée banana, milk, water, and protein powder.
2. Coarsely chop the nuts. Rinse and dry fresh blueberries (or thaw and drain excess liquid from frozen blueberries.)
3. Pour banana-coconut milk mixture into a breakfast bowl. Add blueberries and garnish with nuts and coconut flakes.
4. Add 1 tsp of honey if desired.

FRUIT BELLY

- 4 oz steamed carrots
- 4 oz steamed beets
- ½ cup coconut milk
- 1 oz gelatin (instant)
- Water or ice cubes (optional)

EASY TO VARY – ALTERNATIVE RECIPES ON THE NEXT PAGE

Preparation:
1. Mix all ingredients using an immersion blender or blender.
2. If the smoothie is too thick, add some water or ice cubes to reach the desired consistency.
3. Drink immediately or pour it into a bottle to take-away.

BEET/CARROT SMOOTHIE

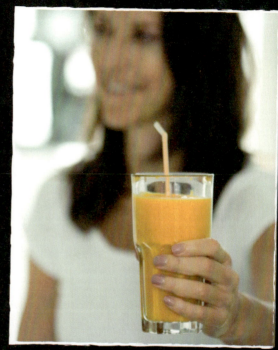

 PREPARATION TIME: 10 MINS

 INGREDIENTS FOR 1 SERVING

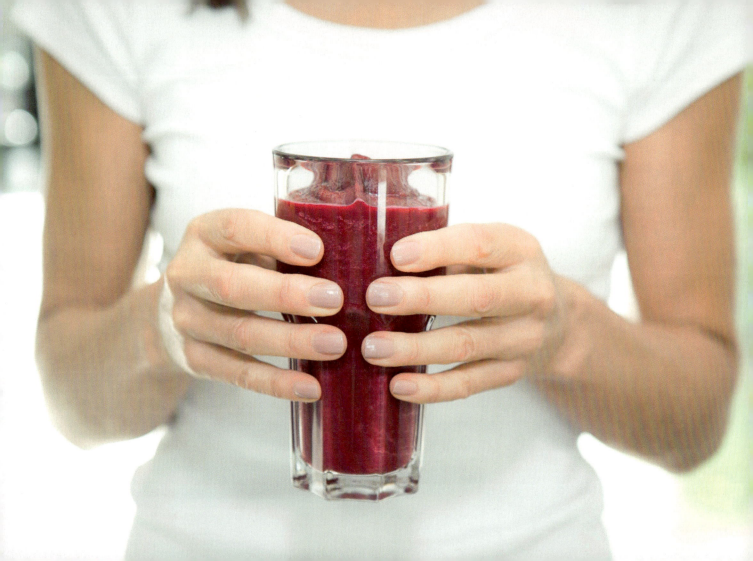

DELICIOUS, HEALTHY, AND REALLY EASY TO MAKE

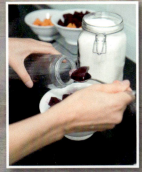
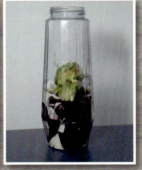
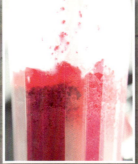
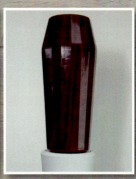
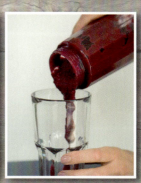

CARROT/COCONUT MILK SMOOTHIE

- ¾ lb steamed beets
- 3 oz avocado
- 1 gelatin (instant)
- Pinch of sea salt
- Water or ice cubes (optional)
- Pinch of cardamom or cinnamon (optional)

Preparation:
Same as the Beet/Carrot Smoothie on page 137

BEET/AVOCADO SMOOTHIE

- ¾ lb steamed beets
- 3 oz avocado
- 1 gelatin (instant)
- Pinch of sea salt
- Water or ice cubes (optional)

Preparation:
Same as the Beet/Carrot Smoothie on page 137

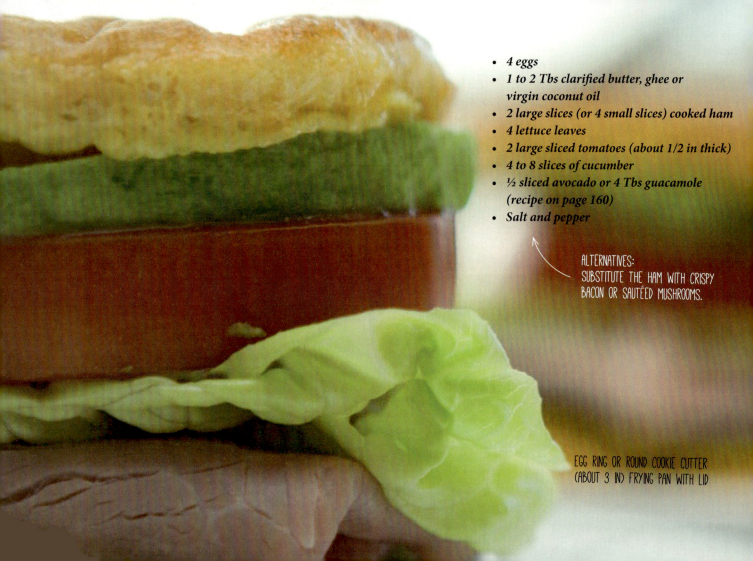

- 4 eggs
- 1 to 2 Tbs clarified butter, ghee or virgin coconut oil
- 2 large slices (or 4 small slices) cooked ham
- 4 lettuce leaves
- 2 large sliced tomatoes (about 1/2 in thick)
- 4 to 8 slices of cucumber
- ½ sliced avocado or 4 Tbs guacamole (recipe on page 160)
- Salt and pepper

ALTERNATIVES: SUBSTITUTE THE HAM WITH CRISPY BACON OR SAUTÉED MUSHROOMS.

EGG RING OR ROUND COOKIE CUTTER (ABOUT 3 IN) FRYING PAN WITH LID

Preparation:
1. Whisk the eggs in individual bowls, season with salt and pepper.
2. Grease the egg ring with clarified butter.
3. Melt some clarified butter in a non-stick frying pan on medium heat. Carefully place the egg ring in the pan and gently hold it in place with one hand.
4. Pour the whisked egg into the egg ring. Hold the egg ring down for another 15 seconds so that no egg will leak out from the bottom.
5. Put the lid on the pan and cook for 5 to 7 minutes. Reduce heat if necessary, so that the omelette will not get too brown on the bottom.
6. Once the omelette is firm on the top, carefully slide the egg ring onto a plate. Using a knife, carefully cut along the edge of the egg ring to release the omelette. Remove the egg ring and set aside, keeping warm.
7. Repeat with the remaining eggs. After all omelettes are done, lightly sauté the sliced tomatoes in the remaining ghee or clarified butter, using the same frying pan.
8. To assemble the burgers: Place one omelette in the middle of the plate as the bottom "bun." Then layer the lettuce leaves, sliced tomatoes, ham, cucumber slices, and avocado (or guacamole). Finally place an omelette on top as the "bun."

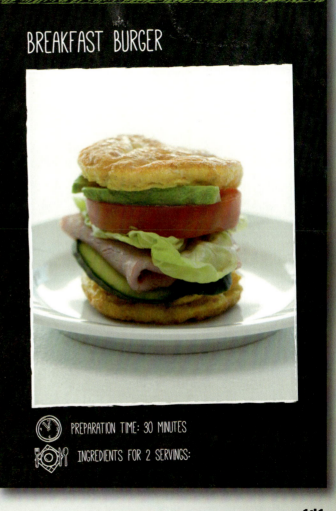

BREAKFAST BURGER

PREPARATION TIME: 30 MINUTES

INGREDIENTS FOR 2 SERVINGS:

BUTTER COFFEE (HOT)

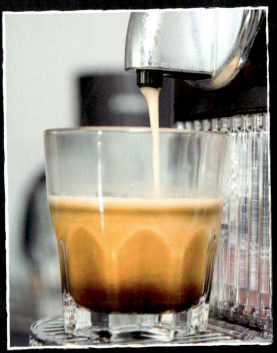

 PREPARATION TIME: 5 MINUTES

 INGREDIENTS FOR 1 SERVING

- 1 coffee or espresso (hot)
- ¾ oz organic raw milk butter (or organic butter or virgin coconut oil)
- Boiling water

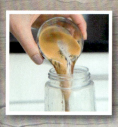 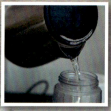 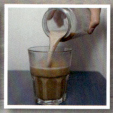

Preparation:
1. Mix coffee and butter in blender for about 30 seconds until the coffee is creamy and foamy and looks similar to a Latte Macchiato.
2. Pour into a glass or mug and add boiling water to taste.

- 1 coffee or espresso (hot)
- ¾ oz organic raw milk butter (or organic butter or virgin coconut oil)
- Ice cubes

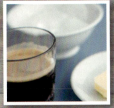 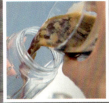 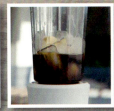

Preparation:
1. Mix hot coffee and butter in blender and blend for about 30 seconds until creamy and foamy.
2. Fill a glass with ice cubes. Pour the hot Butter Coffee over the ice cubes.

BUTTER COFFEE (COLD)

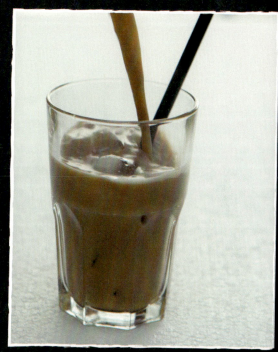

 PREPARATION TIME: 5 MINUTES

 INGREDIENTS FOR 1 SERVING

CHAPTER 6 | RECIPES – BREAKFAST

143

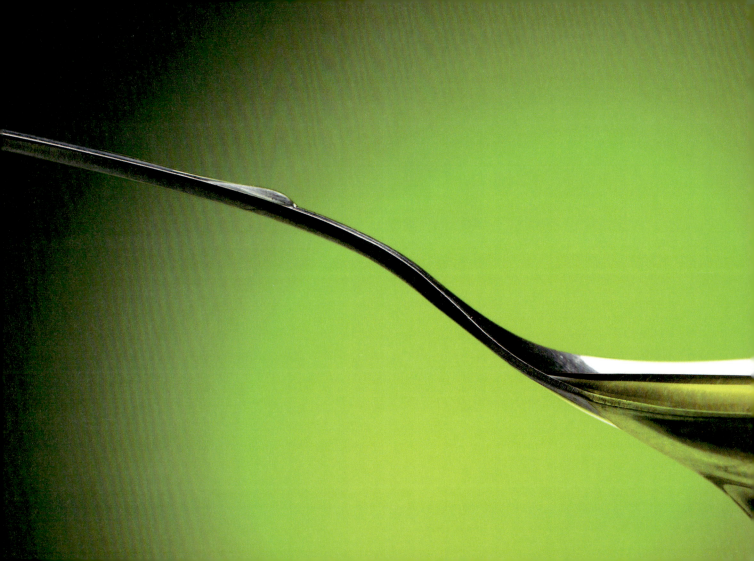

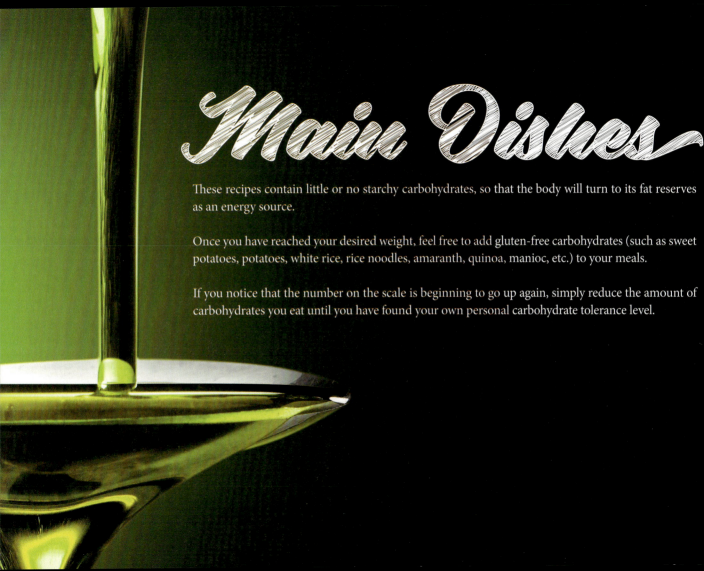

Main Dishes

These recipes contain little or no starchy carbohydrates, so that the body will turn to its fat reserves as an energy source.

Once you have reached your desired weight, feel free to add gluten-free carbohydrates (such as sweet potatoes, potatoes, white rice, rice noodles, amaranth, quinoa, manioc, etc.) to your meals.

If you notice that the number on the scale is beginning to go up again, simply reduce the amount of carbohydrates you eat until you have found your own personal carbohydrate tolerance level.

- 2 large zucchini
- ¾ lb cooked and peeled shrimps
- ¼ lb cherry tomatoes (optional)
- ¼ lb spinach leaves (optional)
- 1 bunch fresh coriander
- 1 small red chili (optional)
- 2 Tbs clarified butter, ghee or olive oil
- 1 Tbs tamari (gluten free soy sauce)
- 1 Tbs lemon juice
- Sea salt
- Pepper

ALTERNATIVE: SUBSTITUTE SHRIMP WITH FRESH, FINELY CHOPPED SALMON.

ALTERNATIVE: INSTEAD OF USING SHRIMP, GARNISH THE ZOODLES WITH CRUMBLED FETA (SHEEP/GOAT'S MILK).

Preparation:

1. Rinse and dry the zucchini, tomatoes, spinach, coriander, and chili.
2. Cut the ends off the zucchini and cut it into long, thin strips with a spiralizer, julienne peeler or vegetable peeler.
3. Slice the chili into fine strips. Pluck the coriander leaves from the stems. Halve the cherry tomatoes.
4. Heat the butter or oil in a frying pan and sauté the zucchini noodles (zoodles) and add chili. Stir gently so that the zoodles cook evenly. After about 2 minutes, add the shrimp, spinach, and tomatoes. Sauté for 2 to 3 minutes until the spinach wilts and the shrimps are warm.
5. Drizzle with tamari and lemon juice and season with salt and pepper if necessary. Add coriander and arrange on plates.

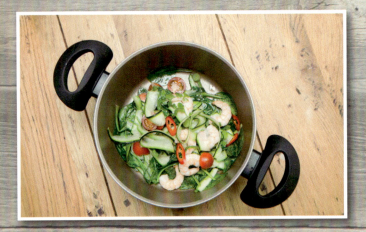

FRUIT BELLY

Zoodles with Shrimp

PREPARATION TIME: 30 MINUTES   INGREDIENTS FOR 2 SERVINGS

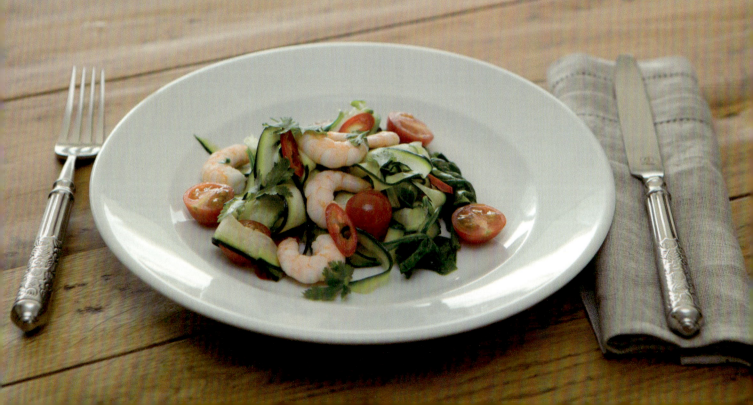

RECIPES—MAIN DISHES

SASHIMI PUZZLE

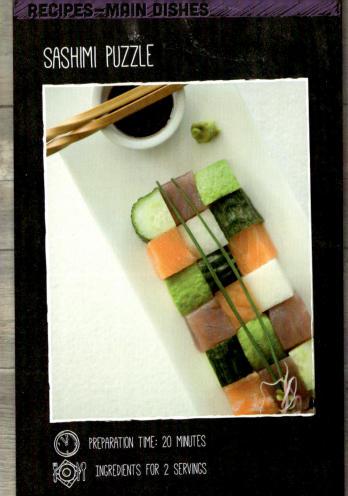

PREPARATION TIME: 20 MINUTES
INGREDIENTS FOR 2 SERVINGS

- ¼ lb fresh salmon (sashimi quality)
- ¼ lb fresh tuna (sashimi quality)
- ½ lb cucumber
- ¼ lb kohlrabi or radish (raw)
- 1 avocado
- Radish sprouts (optional)
- Fresh chives (optional)
- 1 sheet of nori, finely chopped (optional)
- Wasabi paste (gluten-free)
- Tamari (gluten free soy sauce)

Preparation:
1. Rinse and dry the cucumber. Peel kohlrabi or radish. Cut avocado in half, remove the pit and take off the peel.
2. Cut all ingredients into equally sized cubes (about ½ x ½ inch).
3. Arrange on two plates or platters in a puzzle-like pattern (see picture). Garnish with radish sprouts and thin strips of nori and/or chives.
4. Serve tamari and wasabi paste in small bowls on the side.

- 1 large cucumber
- 1 head of lettuce
- 1 avocado
- 1 bunch of parsley
- 2 Tbs lime or lemon juice
- 1 cup water
- ½ tsp sea salt or flower salt
- Black pepper or cayenne (optional)
- 5 oz feta cheese made from goat's or sheep milk (optional) or
- ½ lb peeled and cooked shrimp

Preparation:
1. Cut avocado in half, remove the pit and take off the peel. Rinse and dry vegetables and herbs.
2. Mix all ingredients, except half of the water and the spices, in a blender, adding more water until the soup is thick and creamy.
3. Season with salt and pepper (and cayenne) and ladle into two bowls. Garnish with feta or shrimp.

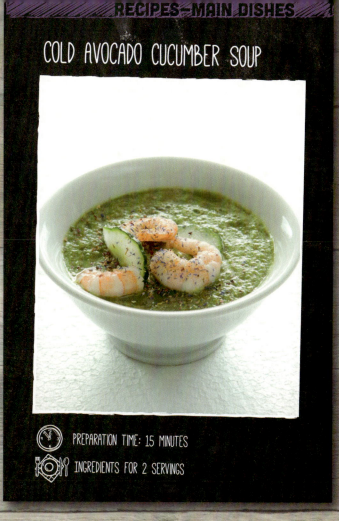

RECIPES—MAIN DISHES

COLD AVOCADO CUCUMBER SOUP

PREPARATION TIME: 15 MINUTES

INGREDIENTS FOR 2 SERVINGS

CHAPTER 6 | RECIPES – MAIN DISHES

Mushroom Kebabs
on Potato and Celeriac Purée

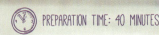 PREPARATION TIME: 40 MINUTES 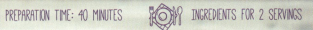 INGREDIENTS FOR 2 SERVINGS

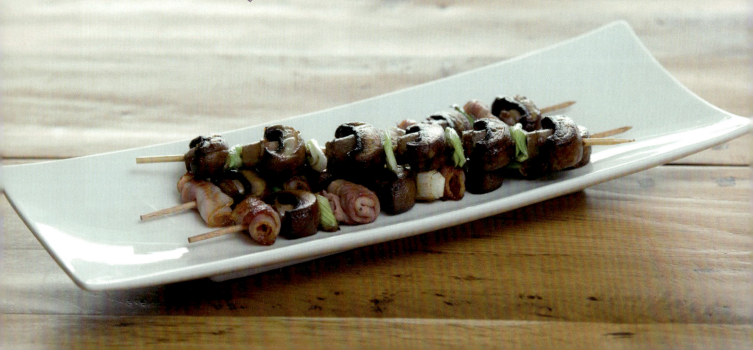

- 4 wooden skewers
- 1 lb mushrooms
- 4 slices of fried bacon (optional)
- 2 slices of boiled ham (optional)
- 1 small onion, peeled,
- 1 Tbs clarified butter or ghee
- 1 bunch parsley, rinsed and finely chopped
- 5 oz peeled celeriac
- 5 oz potatoes, peeled
- ½ cup coconut milk
- Chives, rinsed and diced
- Sea salt
- Pepper

ALTERNATIVES:
SUBSTITUTE MUSHROOMS WITH VEAL, PORK, LAMB, OR CHICKEN.

Preparation:
1. Cut celeriac and potatoes and cook in boiling salt water until tender. Drain salt water, reserving ½ cup for later use. Mix the potatoes and celeriac in a blender with the coconut milk, adding some of the reserved salt water if the purée is too thick. Season with salt and pepper, sprinkle with chives and set aside, keeping it warm.
2. Clean the mushrooms and cut lengthwise in half. Cut onion into eighths, cut bacon in half and roll, cut ham into four pieces and roll. Now stick the mushrooms, onions, ham, and bacon rolls on the skewers.
3. In a large skillet, heat the clarified butter on medium heat and cook the kebabs until browned. Season with salt and pepper and sprinkle with parsley just before taking them out of the pan.
4. Place the skewers on the plate next to or on top of the purée.

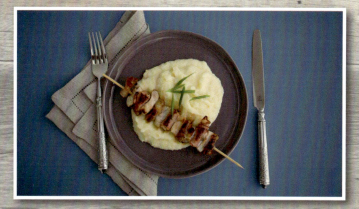

Quick Fix recipe: make skewers with veal or chicken, do not use onions or mushrooms because these can cause flatulence!

CHAPTER 6 | RECIPES – MAIN DISHES

RECIPES—MAIN DISHES

THAI SOUP

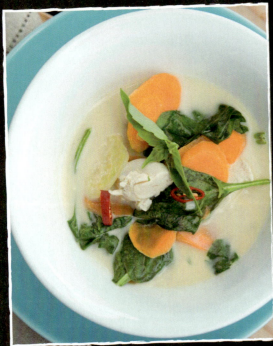

 PREPARATION TIME: 40 MINUTES

 INGREDIENTS FOR 2 PORTIONS:

- ½ lb skinless chicken breasts
- 4 oz fresh spinach
- 1 lb peeled carrots
- 1 cup coconut milk
- 1½ cup water
- 2 stalks lemongrass, outermost shell removed
- 1 oz fresh ginger, peeled
- Fresh chili (optional)
- Fresh (Thai) basil
- Sea salt

Preparation:
1. Rinse spinach and drain. Thinly slice ginger and chili. Cut chicken breasts into pieces. Slice the carrots.
2. Heat water and coconut milk in a pan. Add carrots, ginger, lemongrass, chili and simmer for 20 minutes.
3. Add chicken, spinach and basil, and simmer for another 10 minutes. Season to taste with sea salt and garnish with more fresh basil if desired.
4. Remove the lemongrass stalks before serving.

- ½ lb peeled sweet potatoes
- ½ lb eggplant
- ½ lb zucchini
- ½ lb tuna (canned in water, drained)
- 4 Tbs extra virgin olive oil
- Fresh herbs (basil or chives)
- Sea salt
- Cayenne pepper (optional, very spicy)

ALTERNATIVES: VEGETABLE SALAD CAN ALSO BE EATEN WITH SAUTÉED VEAL OR BEEF CUTLETS, CHICKEN, STEAK OR BURGERS.

Preparation:

1. Preheat oven to 350° F. Line a baking sheet with parchment paper. Cut sweet potatoes, eggplant, and zucchini into equally sized pieces and put on baking sheet. Bake for 20 minutes. Once the roasted vegetables are done, remove and allow to slightly cool.
2. Rinse herbs, pat dry, and chop.
3. Put sweet potatoes, eggplant, zucchini, and herbs in a bowl. Add 2 Tbs olive oil and mix. Season with sea salt and cayenne pepper.
4. Drain the tuna and place in a bowl and mix with 2 Tbs olive oil, salt and pepper.
5. Put the vegetable salad on two plates and top it with a scoop of tuna.

RECIPES—MAIN DISHES

TUNA SALAD WITH VEGETABLES

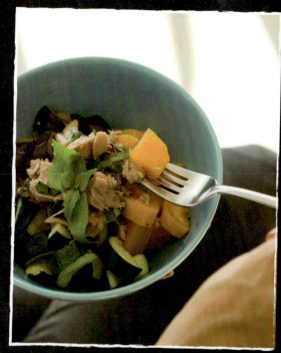

 PREPARATION TIME: 40 MINUTES

 INGREDIENTS FOR 2 SERVINGS

- ¾ lb salmon filet (fresh or thawed)
- 1 Tbs coconut oil
- 1 lb fresh spinach (or 10½ ounces frozen spinach without any additives)
- 1 Tbs clarified butter, ghee or coconut oil
- 1 tsp toasted sesame seeds
- 1 lb cauliflower (rinsed, stem removed, and cut into chunks)
- 1 Tbs olive oil
- Sea salt
- Black pepper and/or cayenne (very spicy)

Preparation:

1. Grate cauliflower chunks in a food processor until it has the consistency of rice.
2. Blanch the cauliflower "rice" in boiling salt water for 2 minutes until it's al dente. Drain and add 1 Tbs olive oil to the "rice," add salt if needed. Cover to keep warm.
3. Wash spinach and slightly drain. Heat butter or oil and add add the spinach. Cover the pan and steam for 2 minutes. Remove lid and finish cooking until the water evaporates. Season well with salt and pepper.
4. Melt 1 Tbs of butter or oil on medium heat and cook the salmon skin side down for about 3 minutes. Flip and continue cooking the other side to desired doneness.
5. Put some "rice" on two plates. Place the spinach on top of or next to it then place half of the salmon filet on each plate. Sprinkle with sesame seeds.

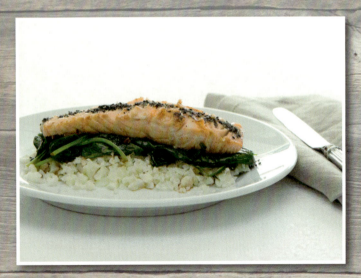

Quick Fix Recipe: Substitute cauliflower rice with 6 oz steamed potatoes

FRUIT BELLY

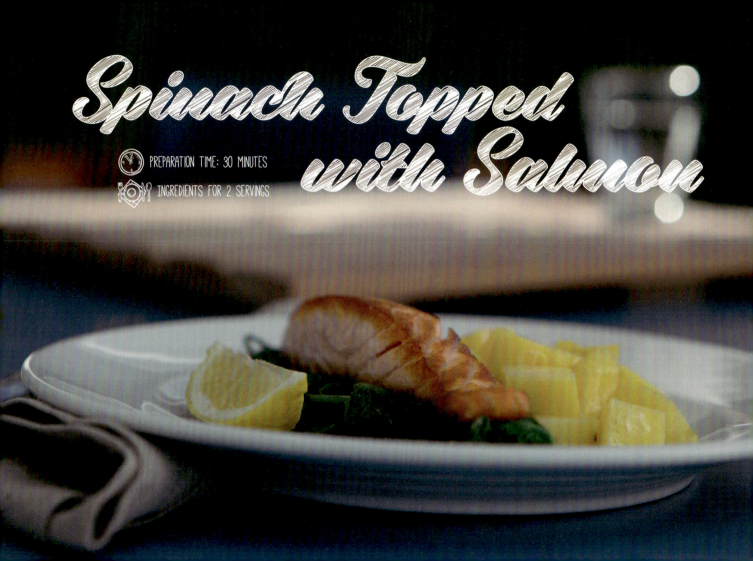

Spinach Topped with Salmon

PREPARATION TIME: 30 MINUTES
INGREDIENTS FOR 2 SERVINGS

RECIPES – MAIN DISHES

CHICKEN BREAST WITH SWEET POTATO AND CARROT SALAD

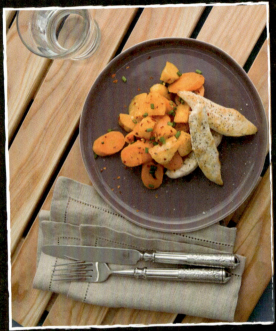

PREPARATION TIME: 30 MINUTES

INGREDIENTS FOR 2 PORTIONS

- ½ lb skinless chicken breasts
- 1 Tbs clarified butter, ghee or coconut oil
- ¾ lb peeled carrots
- ½ lb peeled sweet potatoes
- 3 Tbs extra virgin olive oil
- Sea salt, pepper
- Chili flakes
- Fresh herbs (parsley, tarragon)

Preparation:
1. Cut carrots and sweet potatoes into equally sized pieces. Cook in salt water or in steamer. Allow to cool in a bowl after cooking.
2. Melt 1 Tbs of ghee in a frying pan over medium heat and sauté the chicken on both sides. Reduce heat and cover pan, allow to cook until done.
3. Finely chop the herbs and add to the vegetables. Add olive oil and chili flakes and carefully toss together. Season with sea salt and pepper.

GROUND BEEF AND TOMATO STEW

- 10 oz ground beef (not lean!)
- 14 oz peeled tomatoes, chopped (or non-seasoned canned tomatoes)
- 1 cup water
- ½ lb peeled and cut potatoes
- Fresh basil, parsley, thyme, and/or oregano
- Dried herbs (optional)
- Sea salt, pepper
- Cayenne pepper (optional, very spicy)

Preparation:
1. Sauté ground beef in non-stick pan over medium heat. Add tomatoes and ½ cup of water. Season with salt and pepper. Simmer for 15 minutes.
2. Rinse herbs, pat dry, and chop. Add the herbs and potatoes to the meat and tomatoes and continue to cook until potatoes are done (about 20 minutes depending on the size of the potato pieces).
3. Season with salt and pepper to taste.

Note: If there is only lean beef available, use ghee or clarified butter to sauté the beef.

PREPARATION TIME: 40 MINUTES

INGREDIENTS FOR 2 SERVINGS

Cauliflower Steak

with Poached Eggs and Sweet Potato Fries

PREPARATION TIME: 40 MINUTES

INGREDIENTS FOR 2 SERVINGS

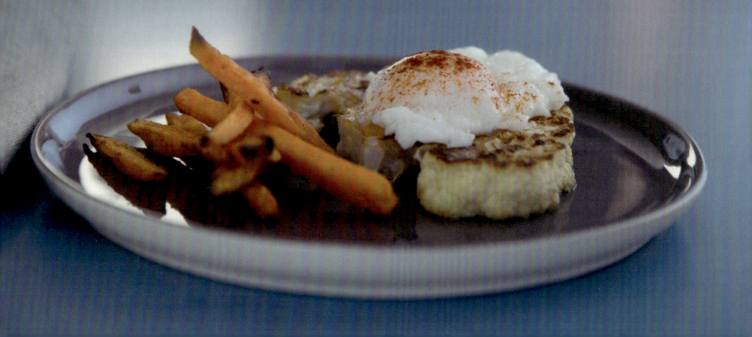

- 1 large cauliflower
- 4 eggs
- 1 lb peeled sweet potatoes
- 3 Tbs coconut oil
- Sea salt
- Cayenne pepper (very spicy) and/or paprika

ALTERNATIVE: SUBSTITUTE THE POACHED EGGS WITH SUNNY SIDE UP EGGS

Preparation:
1. Preheat the oven to 350° F. Put the baking sheet in the oven so that it will get really hot.
2. Cut sweet potatoes lengthwise into equally thick strips. Melt 2 Tbs of coconut oil. Put the fries in a large bowl and pour the coconut oil over them. Add salt and pepper and sprinkle with paprika (cayenne). Using your hands, mix the fries, oil, and spices together until fries are evenly coated.
3. Carefully take the baking sheet out of the oven. Put parchement paper on the sheet and spread the fries in a single layer. Bake for 20 minutes.
4. Remove leaves from the cauliflower. Using a large knife, and starting from the middle of the cauliflower, cut two large slices, about ½ inch thick.
5. Heat 1 Tbs of coconut oil in a frying pan and sauté the cauliflower "steaks" on both sides until lightly browned.
6. Carefully remove cauliflower from the pan so that the slices remain whole. Place on the sheet next to the sweet potatoes. Turn the fries so that they will be evenly brown and crispy. Bake for another 10 to 15 minutes until cauliflower is done.
7. Bring the water to a boil. Crack the eggs individually into a bowl and, depending on the size of the pan, gently slide the eggs into the boiling water one at a time. Reduce heat immediately, so that the water is only slightly simmering. Allow the eggs to cook 3 to 5 minutes depending on the desired consistency of the egg yolk. Using a slotted spoon, take the eggs carefully out of the water.
8. Place two poached eggs on top of each cauliflower steak and season with salt, pepper, and paprika. Serve with the sweet potato fries.

- ¾ lb ground chicken or turkey
- 2 spring onions
- 2 Tbs dijon mustard
- 2 slices of zucchini (see photo)
- 1 ripe avocado
- ½ bunch fresh chives
- 1 tsp sambal oelek (raw chili paste)
- 4 strips bacon
- Lettuce leaves
- ¾ oz Parmesan or Pecorino (lactose-free)
- Salad and sliced pickles
- Sea salt
- Black pepper
- 2 servings of sweet potato fries (see recipe on page 159)

4. Cut the avocado in half and remove the pit. Scoop avocado into a bowl. Rinse chives and chop. Add chives, sambal oelek, pepper and salt to the avocado and mash together.
5. Fry the bacon on both sides until crispy and brown. Carefully remove from the pan, allow to drain on paper towels.
6. Using the bacon grease, fry the burgers and zucchini slices. Make sure that the chicken/turkey burgers are completely cooked through, this takes about 10 minutes, depending on the thickness of the burgers.
7. Grate the cheese.
8. Place the zucchini slices on the plates, layer with the burger, bacon, pickles, and lettuce. Put a scoop of guacamole on top of the lettuce and garnish with cheese.
9. Serve with sweet potato fries and the remaining guacamole on the side.

Preparation:
1. Rinse spring onions, discarding the roots and most of the green part. Finely chop.
2. Mix the ground meat, chopped onion, mustard, salt and pepper in a bowl. The best way to do this is to use your hands.
3. Make two burgers from the meat mixture, making a slight indentation in the middle so that they will cook evenly.

Only use very ripe avocados when making guacamole. You'll know when the avocado is ripe when it is soft to the touch.

Paleo Burger

PREPARATION TIME: 40 MINUTES **INGREDIENTS FOR 2 SERVINGS**

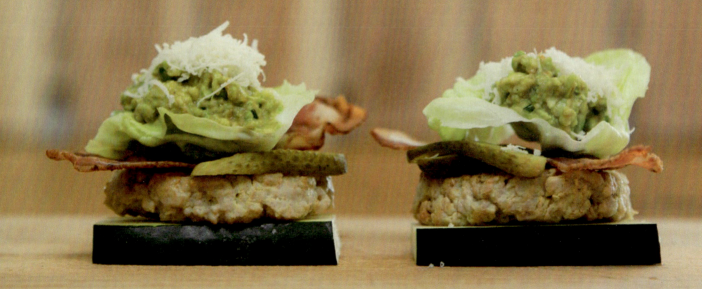

RECIPES—MAIN DISHES

SWEET POTATO NOODLES WITH CHICKEN LIVER

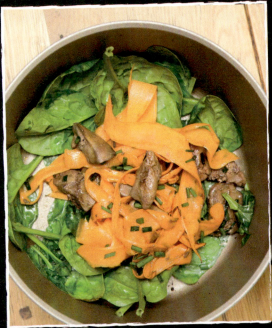

 PREPARATION TIME: 40 MINUTES

 INGREDIENTS FOR 2 SERVINGS

- 1 Tbs butter
- ½ bunch fresh chives
- Sea salt
- Black pepper or cayenne (very spicy)
- 1 lb peeled sweet potatoes
- 2 Tbs clarified butter, ghee or coconut oil
- ½ lb fresh spinach, rinsed and dried

ALTERNATIVES: SUBSTITUTE THE CHICKEN LIVERS WITH THINLY SLICED VEAL, BEEF, OR PORK CUTLETS. SUBSTITUE THE CHICKEN LIVERS WITH PRAWNS WRAPPED IN BACON. SUBSTITUTE THE CHICKEN LIVERS WITH 2 POACHED OR SUNNY SIDE UP EGGS.

Preparation:

1. Rinse chicken liver under cold water and pat dry with paper towels. Trim away the membranes, fibers, and fat.
2. Rinse chives and pat dry. Chop.
3. Cut sweet potatoes with a vegetable slicer or peeler into long thin strips.
4. Lightly fry the liver in a preheated nonstick pan (without any added butter or oil) for 1 to 2 minutes per side.
5. Turn off the heat and add 1 Tbs of butter to the liver. Sprinkle with chives, salt and pepper, set aside, and keep warm.
6. Heat the clarified butter in a large frying pan on medium-high heat and sauté the sweet potato noodles until done. Add spinach and cook until wilted. Add salt and pepper.
7. Place the noodles and spinach on two plates. Top with the liver.

PUMPKIN SOUP WITH CHICKEN BREAST

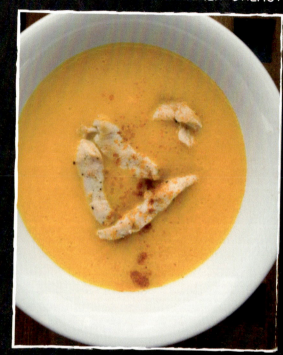

- ½ lb pumpkin, peeled (butternut, muscat or baby bear)
- ½ lb peeled potatoes
- ½ lb skinless chicken breasts
- 1 cup coconut milk
- 1 cup water
- 1 oz fresh ginger, peeled and grated
- Sea salt, pepper
- Ground nutmeg (optional)
- Turmeric (optional)
- Ground cinnamon (optional)

ALTERNATIVE: SUBSTITUTE THE CHICKEN BREAST WITH ½ LB LARGE COOKED AND PEELED SHRIMP.

Preparation:
1. Cut pumpkin and potatoes. Cook in salt water or steamer until done.
2. Cut chicken breasts into thin strips and fry in a non-stick pan. Season with salt and pepper and set aside, keeping warm.
3. Blend coconut milk, water, pumpkin, potatoes, and grated ginger using a blender, food processor or immersion blender. Heat, adding either water or coconut milk if too thick. Season with salt and spices. Add the cooked chicken strips and heat to desired temperature.

 PREPARATION TIME: 30 MINUTES

 INGREDIENTS FOR 2 SERVINGS

- 3 pieces of parchment paper
- 2 fish filets (5 oz fresh or thawed)
- 4 thin slices of lemon
- 2 oz fresh ginger
- 4 large fresh basil leaves
- 1 lb steamed and peeled beets
- 2 Tbs olive oil
- Thyme (fresh and/or dried)
- Sea salt
- Pepper
- 1 oz salted and shelled pistachios

5. Cut the beets into equally sized pieces and place in a bowl. Rinse the thyme and pat dry. Strip leaves from the stems. Add 2 Tbs olive oil, thyme, salt and pepper to the beets and mix well. Place the beets on the other half of the baking sheet.
6. Bake the fish packages and beets for 20 minutes.
7. Place a fish package and half of the beets on each plate. Garnish with pistachios and some more thyme if desired.
8. Beets with pistachios can be eaten cold as a salad. They also make a quick meal along with some canned tuna or smoked trout filet.

Preparation:
1. Preheat the oven to 350° F. Line a large baking sheet with parchment paper.
2. Rinse fish and pat dry. Wash, dry, and cut lemon into thin slices. Peel and slice ginger. Rinse the basil leaves and pat dry.
3. Place two slices of lemon in the middle of each piece of parchment paper. Lay the fish filet on top of the lemon slices and season with salt and pepper. Add the ginger slices and basil.
4. Now fold the parchment paper so that the fish and ingredients are well packed and no steam can escape. Place the fish packages on one side of the baking sheet.

Quick Fix Recipe: Omit pistachios

Fish "Packages"
with Beet Salad

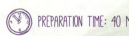 PREPARATION TIME: 40 MINUTES   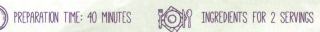 INGREDIENTS FOR 2 SERVINGS

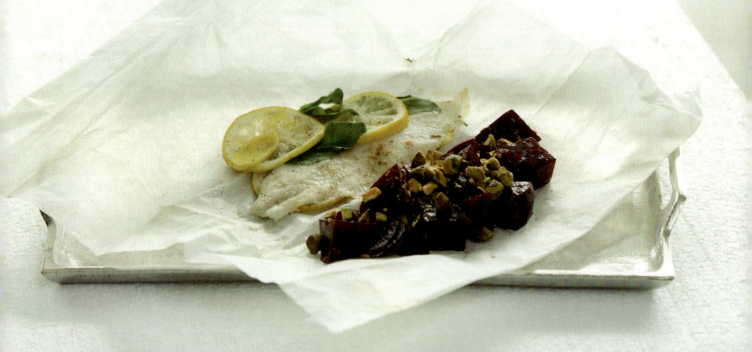

Paleo Bibimbap

 PREPARATION TIME: 40 MINUTES 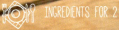 INGREDIENTS FOR 2 SERVINGS

- ½ lb thinly sliced beef, veal, or pork
- 2 Tbs coconut oil
- 2 oz lettuce
- 4 oz carrots
- ½ lb mushrooms
- 1 lb cauliflower (rinsed, stem removed and cut into chunks)
- 2 egg yolks
- Tamari (gluten free soy sauce)
- Fish sauce (optional)
- Tabasco or chili sauce (optional)
- Fresh coriander and/or chives
- Sea salt
- Black pepper and/or cayenne (very spicy)

ALTERNATIVE: SUBSTITUTE THE RAW EGG YOLK WITH A SUNNY SIDE UP OR POACHED EGG.

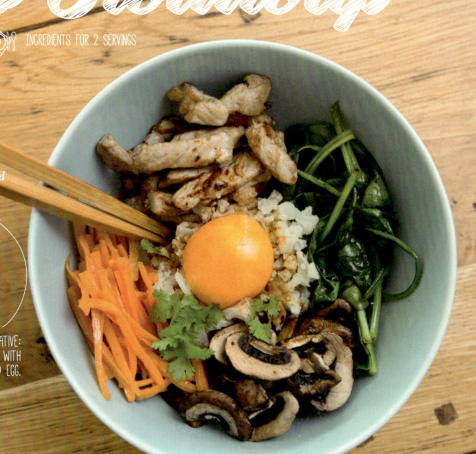

Preparation:

1. Grate cauliflower chunks in a food processor until it has the consistency of rice.
2. Blanch the cauliflower "rice" in boiling salt water for 2 minutes until it's al dente.
3. Drain and add 1 Tbs coconut oil to the "rice" in the pan and season with salt to taste. Cover to keep warm.
4. Peel carrots and cut into thin strips. Rinse spinach and dry. Clean the mushrooms and cut into quarters. Blanch carrots and sauté the mushrooms separately.
5. Slice the meat into thin strips. Heat 1 Tbs of coconut oil in a frying pan and sauté for 1 to 2 minutes. Remove from the pan and keep warm.
6. In the same frying pan, using the remaining coconut oil, sauté the spinach until wilted.
7. Preheat two heat resistant bowls. Put the cauliflower rice in the bowls. Put the hot vegetables and meat on top of the rice, leaving space in the middle for the egg yolk. Carefully place the egg yolk in the center of the bowl.
8. Garnish with fresh coriander and drizzle with tamari, fish sauce, and/or tabasco.

This is how to eat Bibimbap:
At the table, everyone can add more tamari, tabasco, and/or chili sauce and seasonings if desired. Using chopsticks, mix the egg yolk with the "rice." The egg will lightly cook due to the heat of the dish.

Cauliflower rice can also be cooked in the microwave.

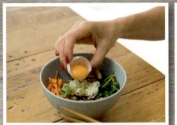 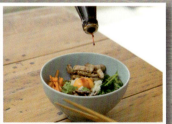 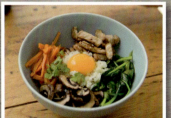 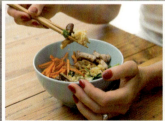

Small Pure Food Paleo Desserts

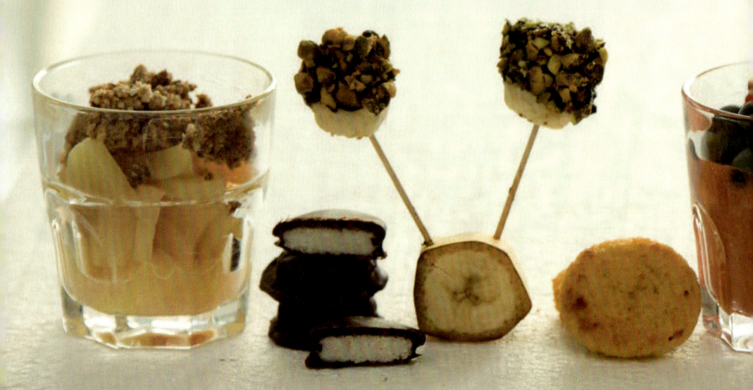

Can you eat dessert and still lose weight? This seems like a contradiction, doesn't it? Well, yes and no. You can't eat a huge, sugar-bomb of a dessert and still lose those pounds. But here you'll find some small desserts made mainly of protein, vegetables, and natural fats that will satisfy your sweet tooth after a meal without having to feel guilty. Food must not only contain all the essential nutrients, but it should also satisfy all the senses. Only by eating the right kind of food will you be able to change your diet and lifestyle for the long-term and successfully maintain your optimal weight.

P.S. If you notice that you are eating more than the recommended portions, or if you are craving more and more sweets, then it might be wise to completely cut out all sweets from your diet for two to three weeks. This should do the trick to break the "sweet" habit.

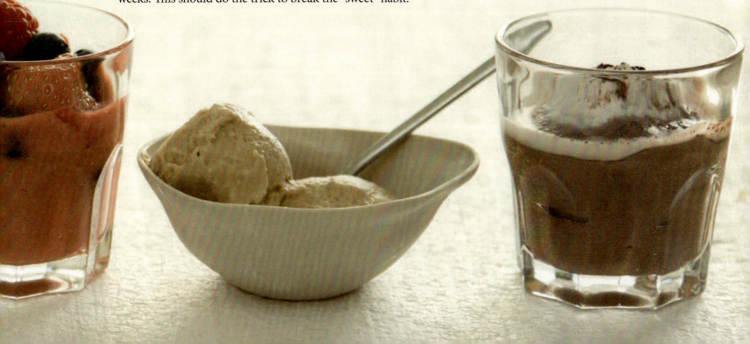

RECIPES—DESSERTS

CHOCOLATE MOUSSE

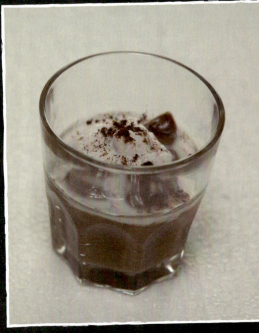

PREPARATION TIME: 10 MINUTES
COOLING TIME: AT LEAST 3 HOURS
INGREDIENTS FOR 2 SERVINGS

- 2 eggs
- 2 oz chocolate (containing at least 70 percent cocoa)
- 1 small pinch of sea salt (optional)

Preparation:
1. Separate the egg whites from the yolks. Whisk the egg whites with a pinch of salt until stiff.
2. Melt the chocolate in a bowl placed over a hot water bath or in the microwave. Add the melted chocolate to the egg yolks stirring constantly.
3. Add one third of the stiff egg whites to the chocolate/egg yolk mixture.
4. Carefully fold the remaining egg whites into the mixture using a spatula.
5. Pour into two glasses or bowls, cover with plastic wrap, and refrigerate for at least 3 hours.

Serving suggestions:
Top the mousse with fresh or stewed berries, whipped coconut cream (or whipped cream).

Please note:
Since raw eggs are used, consume on the same day. Only use fresh eggs.

RECIPES – DESSERTS

APPLE TOPPED WITH CRUMBLE

- 1 large apple
- 1 tsp lemon juice
- 1 Tbs water
- 2 oz almonds, finely ground
- 1 tsp honey
- 1 Tbs coconut oil or butter, melted
- ½ tsp ground cinnamon

ALTERNATIVES:
SUBSTITUTE THE APPLE WITH PEAR OR STONE FRUITS
SUBSTITUTE THE ALMONDS WITH PECANS OR MACADAMIA NUTS.

Preparation:
1. Preheat oven to 350° F. Line a baking sheet with parchment paper.
2. Peel, core, and slice apple. In a small pan, cook with the lemon juice and water for 10 minutes.
3. In a bowl, combine the almonds, honey, coconut oil, and cinnamon, mixing with your fingers until it forms a crumbly mass.
4. Spread the mixture on the baking sheet and bake 7 to 10 minutes until golden brown.
5. Pour the apple sauce into small glasses or bowls and sprinkle with the nut crumble mixture.

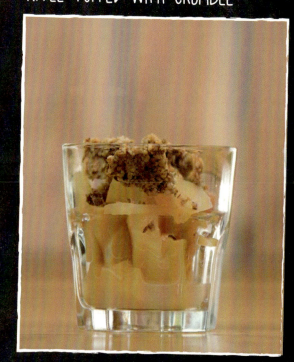

 PREPARATION TIME: 30 MINUTES

 INGREDIENTS FOR 2 SERVINGS

RECIPES—DESSERTS

BANANA CRUNCH

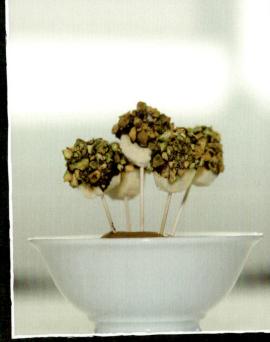

 PREPARATION TIME: 15 MINUTES

 INGREDIENTS FOR 2 SERVINGS

- *1 banana*
- *2 oz chocolate (containing at least 70 percent cocoa)*
- *2 oz salted pistachios*

Preparation:
1. Finely chop pistachios. Melt chocolate in a bowl placed over a hot water bath or in the microwave.
2. Peel the banana and slice into ⅜-inch thick slices. Stick each slice on a wooden skewer stick, dip into the melted chocolate. and then dip into the chopped pistachios.
3. Put banana skewers in the freezer until the chocolate sets, or else eat immediately.

RECIPES—DESSERTS

PALEO BOUNTIES

- 2 oz chocolate (containing at least 70 percent cocoa)
- 1 Tbs coconut oil
- ¾ oz instant gelatin or protein powder (neutral or vanilla flavor)
- ¾ oz desiccated coconut
- 1 Tbs coconut milk

Preparation:
1. Mix desiccated coconut, gelatin, and coconut milk. Shape into four equally sized "bars" and put in the freezer.
2. Melt chocolate and coconut oil in a small bowl placed over a hot water bath, or in the microwave.
3. Dip the chilled coconut pieces into the melted chocolate and put them back into the freezer. Keep the chocolate warm. After 10 minutes, dip the bounties in the chocolate again and put in the fridge to set.
4. Once the chocolate is set, the bounties can be eaten.

These can be stored in the refrigerator for up to a week.

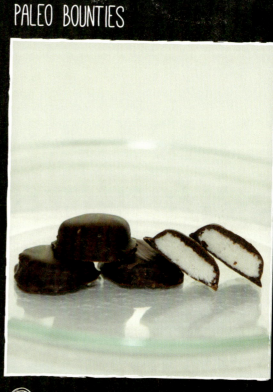

 PREPARATION TIME: 20 MINUTES; COOLING TIME: 30 MINUTES

 INGREDIENTS FOR 2 DESSERT/SNACK SERVINGS

Macadamia Nut Cookies

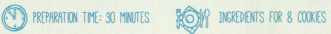 PREPARATION TIME: 30 MINUTES   INGREDIENTS FOR 8 COOKIES

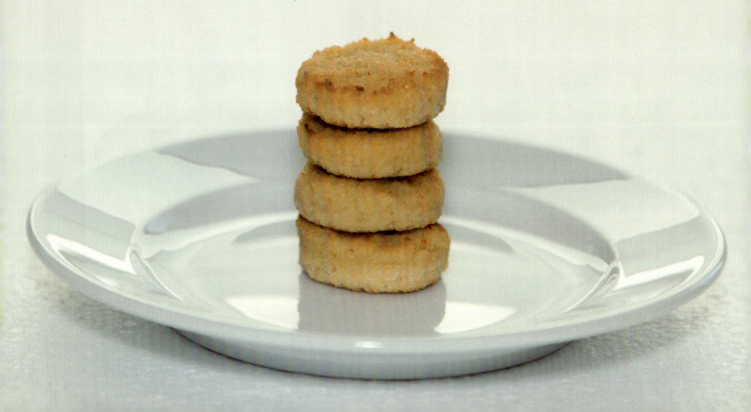

- 3 oz macadamia nuts
- ¾ oz instant gelatine or protein powder (neutral or vanilla flavor)
- 1 egg
- 1 Tbs honey (liquid)
- 1 pinch of salt
- 1 oz desiccated coconut
- ¾ oz cocoa nibs or chopped chocolate (containing at least 70 percent cocoa)

Preparation:
1. Preheat the oven to 350° F. Line the baking sheet with parchment paper.
2. Finely grind macadamia nuts. Mix with all ingredients, except chocolate, forming a dough.
3. Once the dough is formed, add chocolate (if desired).
4. Roll dough into 8 balls and place on the baking sheet. Flatten (a little less than ¼ inch thick).
5. Bake 10 minutes until golden brown.

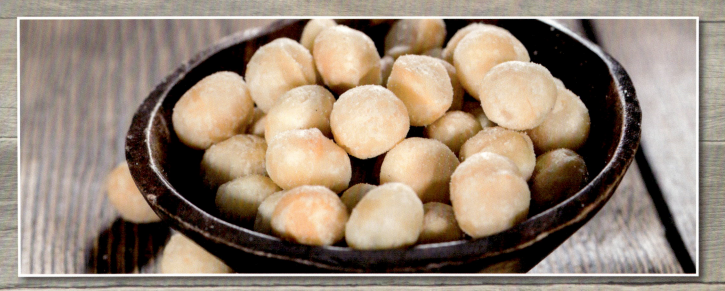

RECIPES—DESSERTS

COFFEE ICE CREAM

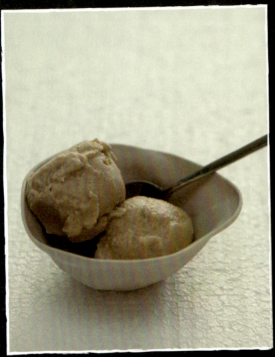

 PREPARATION TIME: 30 MINUTES

INGREDIENTS FOR 4 SERVINGS

- *1 cup coconut milk, cold*
- *1 decaffinated espresso, cooled*
- *1 Tbs honey (liquid)*

Preparation:
1. Mix all ingredients in a blender and pour into an ice cream maker (following the instuctions for the ice cream maker). This will take about 20 minutes.
2. Scoop into bowls and enjoy immediately or freeze for later.
3. Can be decorated with cocoa nibs or grated chocolate.

RECIPES–DESSERTS

BERRY SOUP

- ½ lb fresh or thawed berries
- ¾ oz instant gelatin or vanilla protein powder
- ½ cup coconut milk
- 1 tsp vanilla powder/extract
- 1 Tbs honey (liquid)

Preparation:
1. Mix all ingredients and half of the berries in blender.
2. Pour into glasses and garnish with the remaining berries.

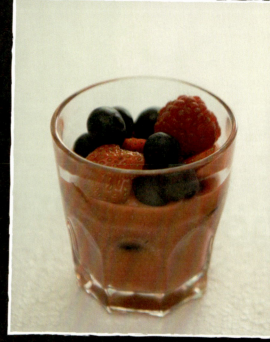

PREPARATION TIME: 5 MINUTES
INGREDIENTS FOR 2 SERVINGS

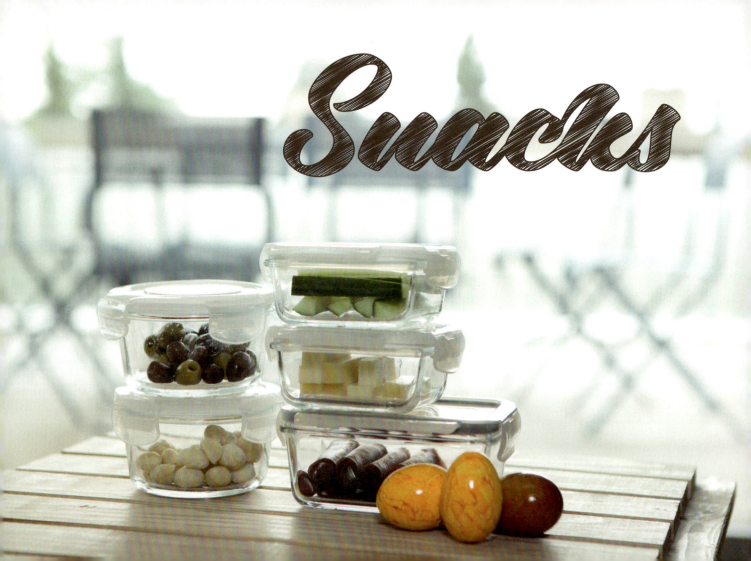

With snacks, it's important that they contain few or no carbohydrates. The danger with snacks containing carbohydrates (like a bar of chocolate) is that they raise blood sugar levels and, after a short time, make us even hungrier than we were before.

A good snack should dampen our hunger level until the next meal. Blood sugar levels should only slightly rise. A snack should relieve hunger signals from our brain to stomach, while still allowing our system to adjust to the dietary change that activates the fat metabolism to give us energy.

RECOMMENDED SNACKS ARE:
One portion consists of one each of the following:
1 oz dried meat (beef jerky or 100 percent natural prosciutto)
1 oz raw milk cheese
1 egg (hard boiled)
1 oz olives
¾ oz macadamia nuts (containing the least amount of carbohydrates of all nuts)

AND

4 oz cucumber or pickles or
4 oz cherry tomatoes

The following snacks are not an option: fruit, carrots, chips, candy, soft drinks, coffee-based drinks sweetened with syrup, all forms of granola bars.

When do I eat a snack? Between the main meals. First drink a glass of water and wait 10 to 20 minutes. If you're still hungry, have a snack. Snacks should not substitute main meals!

How big is a snack?
One portion (see left). A combination of protein and vegetables (such as 1 oz of beef jerky and 4 oz cucumber).

What if I'm still hungry after a snack? Wait 20 minutes, then drink a big glass of water and wait another 10 minutes. If it's not time for a main meal yet, then you may have another snack. If you often seem to be hungry between meals, try making the main meal portions bigger.

The goal is to not need any snacks.
Why is it better to not have any snacks? During the breaks between meals, the body is able to fully and properly digest the food you have eaten. If your body needs energy (and doesn't get a snack) between meals, it will turn to body fat as an energy source.

CHAPTER 6 | RECIPES – SNACKS

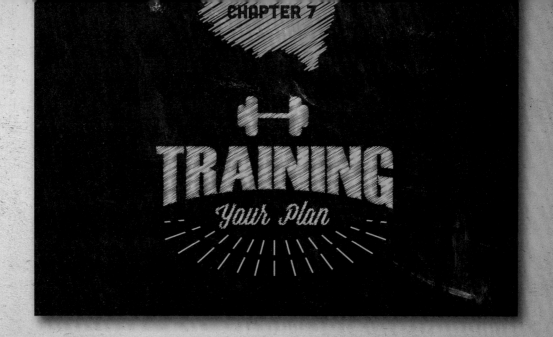

WORKOUT INFORMATION

It's most effective if you exercise intensively on a regular basis.

> **FITNESS IS LIKE MARRIAGE. YOU CAN'T CHEAT ON IT AND EXPECT IT TO WORK.**
> Bonnie Pfiester

You should work out as intensively as you can. It does not depend on your age, gender, or your current fitness level. A 20-year-old woman should take it to the max, and the same goes for a 65-year-old man. Both should work out as intensely as they can, according to their current strength, level of endurance, and flexibility.

HOW OFTEN SHOULD YOU WORK OUT?

- Depending on how much time you have and what your goals are, it's best to work out two to five times a week.
- If you're a beginner, it's best to start with two workouts a week, slowly working your way up to five workouts a week (adding another workout every month), if you can find/make the time.
- It's important to warm up and/or stretch prior to each workout. (see A, B, C, D, E or F on pg. 183).
- Make sure you give yourself recovery time between workouts, 24 to 36 hours should do the trick.
- In addition to your HIIT workouts, you'll want to go for a 30 to 60 minute walk (not jog!) every day.
- You'll want to aim for at least 8,000 steps a day. You could use a pedometer or smart phone app to help you keep track.

Sources for pedometers can be found in Appendix (pg. 215).

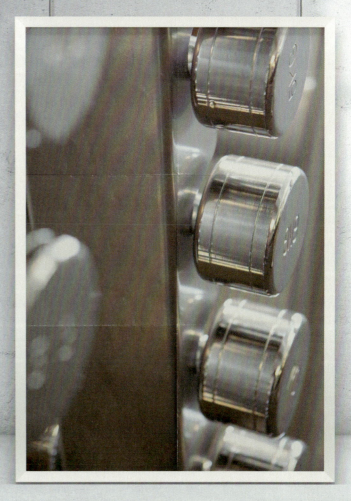

CHAPTER 7 | TRAINING 181

WHY IS PHYSICAL HEALTH SO IMPORTANT?

> **PHYSICAL FITNESS IS NOT ONLY ONE OF THE MOST IMPORTANT KEYS TO A HEALTHY BODY, IT IS THE BASIS OF DYNAMIC AND CREATIVE INTELLECTUAL ACTIVITY.**
>
> John F. Kennedy

A fit body is not only more resistant to disease and stress, a fit body is also more relaxed and can provide more energy for difficult mental tasks.

In an interview with Sir Richard Branson, successful English entrepreneur and billionaire, he was asked how he manages pressure. He said that he was under extreme pressure when his attempts to break the record to sail around the world had failed. Only with a fit body are you able to perform mentally. This is the reason why I keep myself fit.

> **IF YOUR BODY IS SHARP, YOUR BRAIN WILL BE SHARP.**
>
> Sir Richard Branson

WARM UP / LOOSEN UP / STRETCH

	EXERCISE	EQUIPMENT	SETS	INTERVALS	BREAK
A	Cycling (Indoor)	Speed adjustable	8	20 min	10 min
B	Wall sit	Possibly with additional weight	8	20 min	10 min
C	Rowing	Resistance adjustable	8	20 min	10 min
D	Crosstraining	Resistance adjustable	8	20 min	10 min
E	Loosening Muscles	Blackroll		10 to 20 Min.	
F	Stretching			10 to 20 Min.	

10 MINUTE HIIT

EMOTM= every minute on the minute (10 minutes=10 sets)

Men

EXERCISE	EQUIPMENT	1 to 2 min	3 to 4	5 to 6	7 to 8	9 to 10
Push-ups		4	6	8	10	12
Pull-ups	Table, bar	2	4	6	8	10
Thrusters	2 dumbbells or kettlebells	2	4	6	8	10

EMOTM= every minute on the minute (10 minutes=10 sets)

Women

EXERCISE	EQUIPMENT	1 to 2 min	3 to 4	5 to 6	7 to 8	9 to 10
Push-ups		4	6	8	10	12
Squats		4	6	8	10	12
Jumping jacks		8	10	12	14	16

20 MINUTE HIIT

AMSAP= as many sets as possible (20 minutes)

Men & Women

EXERCISE	EQUIPMENT	Set 1	Set 2	Set 3	Set 4	Set 5
Sprints		200 m	100 m	200 m	100 m	200 m
Handstand push-ups	Stairs/bench	5	10	15	20	25
Pull-ups	Table or bar	5	10	15	20	25
Squats		10	20	30	40	50

WARM UP (A, B, C AND D)

A: CYCLING
Program the indoor cycling bike to intervals: 20 seconds high resistance, 10 seconds very low resistance. Repeat this 20/10 second interval 8 times for 4 minutes.

Position: Adjust the seat of your bike so your legs are fully extended when the pedals are at their lowest point.

B: WALL SIT
Position: Actively press your back and buttocks to a wall. Your head, shoulder blades, and lower back should be touching the wall. Thighs and lower legs are at a 90° angle.

Movement: None! This is a static (or isometric) exercise. It's about holding the position for the indicated time.

Alternative to make the exercise more intense: Grab some hand weights and fully extend your arms at shoulder level.

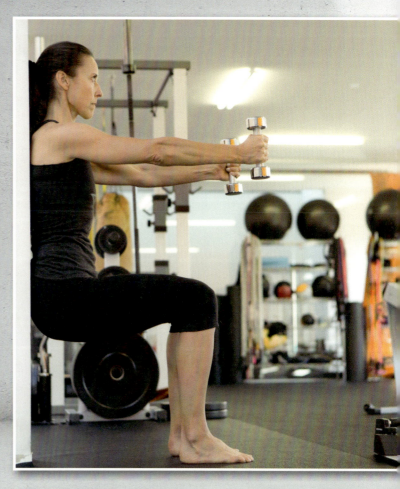

CHAPTER 7 | TRAINING

C: ROWING

Position: Strap your feet in with the straps just below toe level. Sit upright leaning slightly forward, legs bent, arms straight.

Motion: First push your body back with your legs, moving your torso to an upright position. When the legs are nearly fully extended, pull the grip just below chest level using your upper body, leaning slightly back.

Once you've reached this position, push your hands forward past your knees as you bring your body forward, flexing your legs to bring yourself back to the starting position.

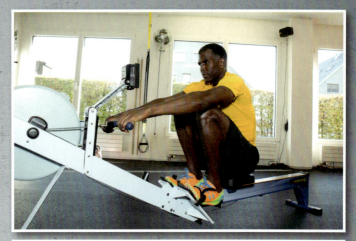

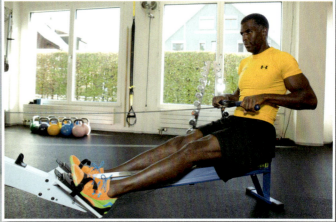

FRUIT BELLY

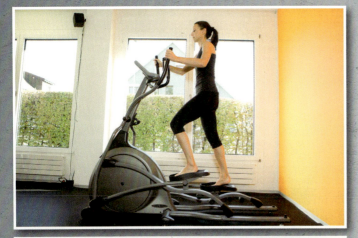

D: CROSSTRAINER

Motion: Keep your body upright during the whole exercise. Roll your steps over the ball of your feet and let your heel move up and down freely.

LOOSENING MUSCLES AND CONNECTIVE TISSUE (E, F, G AND H)

E: THIGHS

Lying on your belly, place a foam roller under your thighs and slowly push yourself forwards and backwards. Turn on your side and repeat the movements, allowing the foam roller to massage the sides of your thighs. Finally, lie on your back, massaging the back of your thighs and calves. Take as much time as you need until your legs are loosened up and relaxed.

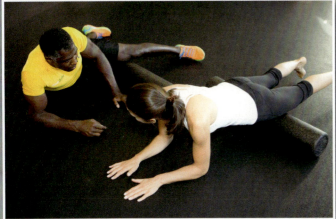

F: UPPER BACK AND SHOULDER BLADES
While lying with your back on the foam roller, fold your arms across your chest und move slowly up and down, working between your shoulder blades. Try the same technique while supporting your head and neck with your hands, keeping your elbows together.

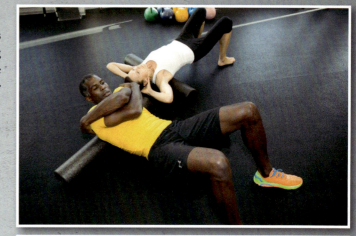

G: BACK MUSCLES
Lying with your back on the foam roller, turn slightly to one side so that you can massage your sides with the foam roller. Keep your hands behind your head while rolling up and down. Repeat on the other side.

To mobilize your upper back, slowly extend both arms up until you touch the floor behind your head, keeping your back on the floor. Take your time and make slow movements. You should not feel any pain. Before long, you will become more and more flexible and will love this stretch.

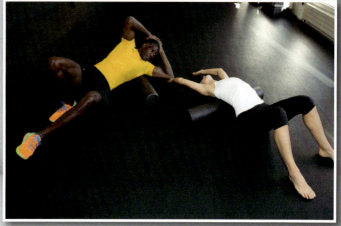

FRUIT BELLY

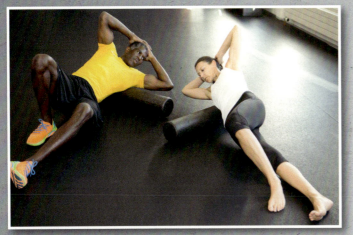

H: LOWER MUSCLES ON YOUR SIDE (WAIST)
Lying on your side, position the roller at waist level. The lower leg should be extended on the floor, the upper leg bent with your foot touching the floor. Support your head with your hands. Using your upper leg to push, gently roll up to shoulder level and down again. At first, this may be a bit painful, but with the support of your top leg, you can adjust the amount of weight on the roller.

STRETCHING (I, J, K, L, M AND N)

I: BACK THIGH AND CALF (OPTION 1)
In a lunge position, bend the upper body forward and slowly extend the front leg. Hold this position and feel your muscles stretch.

J: BACK THIGH AND CALF (OPTION 2)
Downward dog position. Heels are on the floor, legs and arms fully extended. Hands are flat on the floor. Pushing with your arms, your buttocks should be raised up toward the ceiling. Your naval is drawn in towards the spine. Aim for a perfect inverted V-shape.

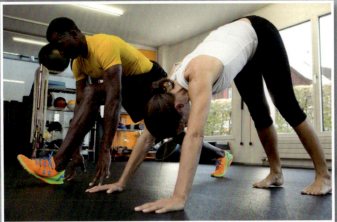

CHAPTER 7 | TRAINING

K: CHEST

Lie with your chest on the floor, one arm stretched out to the side in a 45° angle. Use the other hand to slightly push yourself up off the floor, rotating towards the side where your arm is extended. Feel the stretch in your chest. Repeat on the other side.

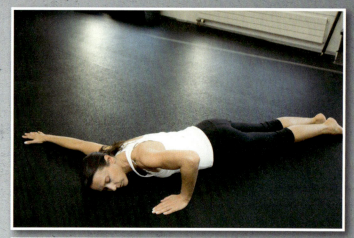

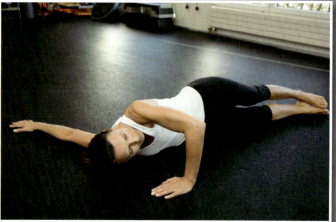

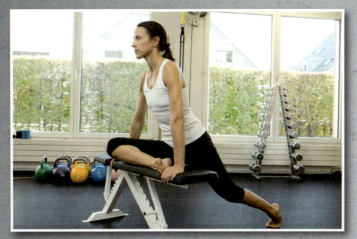

L: BUTTOCKS
Place your lower leg on a bench at a a 90° angle from the lower leg to your upper leg. Lower your hip slowly to increase the stretch. Repeat the exercise with the other leg.

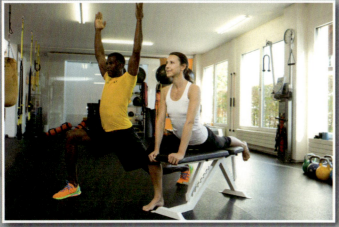

M: HIP FLEXOR (OPTION 1)
Position yourself in a forward lunge, with hands stretched up over your head. Lower your hip until you feel the stretch in your hip flexor. Always keep your upper body straight and your buttocks tight.

N: HIP FLEXOR (OPTION 2)
Lay the front length of one leg on a bench. Keep the foot of your other leg on the floor, bent, as support for your upper body. To increase the stretch you can tighten your buttocks and slowly move your upper body to an upright position.

10-MINUTE HIGH INTENSITY INTERVAL TRAINING (HIIT)

1ST and 2ND ROUND
4 push-ups
2 pull-ups
2 thrusters
Rest 60 seconds

3RD and 4TH ROUND
6 push-ups
4 pull-ups
4 thrusters
Rest 60 seconds

5TH and 6TH ROUND
8 push-ups
6 pull-ups
6 thrusters
Rest 60 seconds

7TH and 8TH ROUND
10 push-ups
8 pull-ups
8 thrusters
Rest 60 seconds

9TH and 10TH ROUND
12 push-ups
10 pull-ups
10 thrusters
Rest 60 seconds

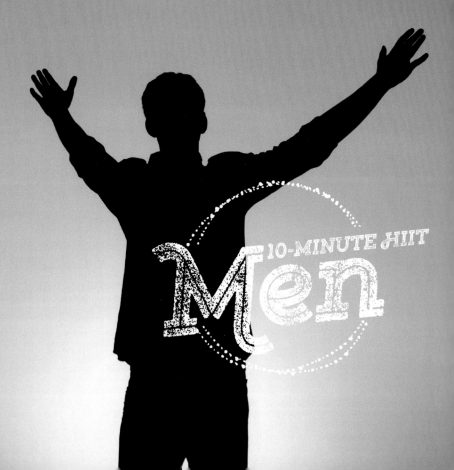

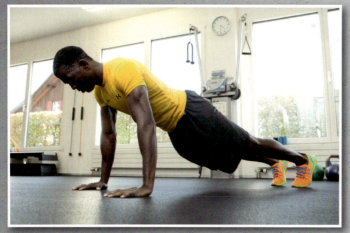

PUSH-UPS

Starting Position: Place your hands slightly wider than shoulders, in line with your chest. Form a straight line with your body from head to toe. Keep your abs and buttocks tight throughout the whole exercise.

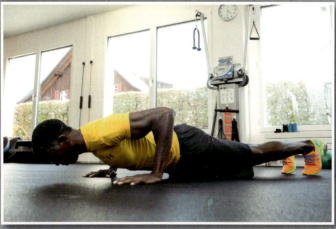

Motion: Bend your arms, lowering yourself to the floor. Touch your chest (sternum) to the floor and push back up until your arms are fully extended.

INVERTED ROW

Starting Position: You can either use a bar positioned at hip level or you can lie under a table. Position yourself, holding on so that you can pull your chest to the bar or the edge of the table. Make sure your body is taut and straight as a board from head to toe.

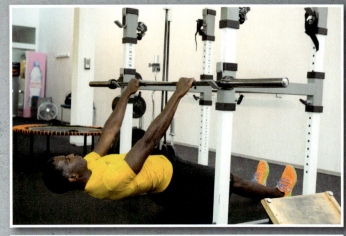

Motion: Pull up until you touch the bar/edge of the table with your chest, keeping your body taut.

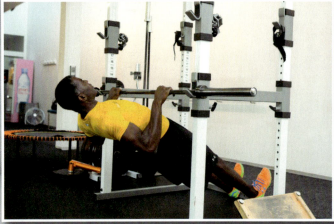

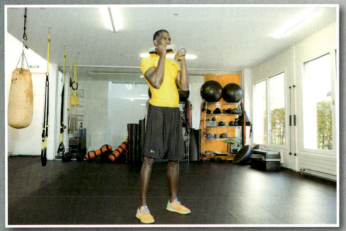

THRUSTERS

Starting position: Stand with your feet parallel, shoulder-width apart. Hold the dumbbells up at shoulder height.

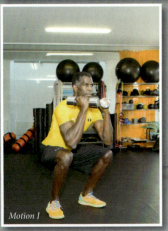
Motion I

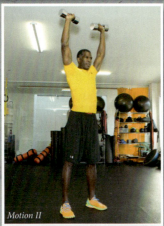
Motion II

Motion I: Squat down with a straight back until your hips are at knee level or lower.

Motion II: Push up with your legs as hard as you can. Once at the starting position, use the momentum to press the dumbbells over your head until your arms are fully extended. Tense your whole body for a short moment, making sure you are in control of the weights. Then lower the dumbbells back to the starting position.

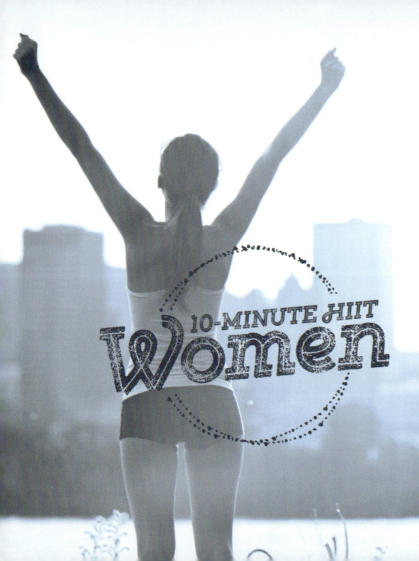

10-MINUTE HIGH INTENSITY INTERVAL TRAINING (HIIT)

1ST and 2ND ROUND
4 push-ups
4 squats
8 jumping jacks
Rest 60 seconds

3RD and 4TH ROUND
6 push-ups
6 pull-ups
10 jumping jacks
Rest 60 seconds

5TH and 6TH ROUND
8 push-ups
8 squats
12 jumping jacks
Rest 60 seconds

7TH and 8TH ROUND
10 push-ups
10 squats
14 jumping jacks
Rest 60 seconds

9TH and 10TH ROUND
12 push-ups
12 squats
16 jumping jacks
Rest 60 seconds

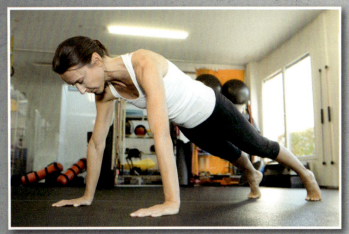

PUSH-UPS

Starting Position: Place your hands slightly wider than shoulders, in line with your chest. Form a straight line with your body from head to toe. Keep your abs and buttocks tight throughout the whole exercise.

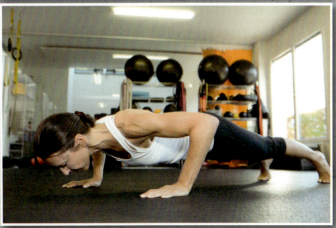

Motion: Bend your arms, lowering yourself to the floor. Touch your chest (sternum) to the floor and push back up until your arms are fully extended.

Easier Alternative:

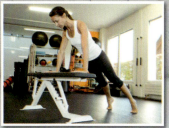
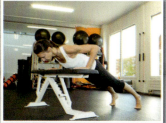

SQUAT

Starting Position: Stand straight with your feet parallel and hip-width apart.

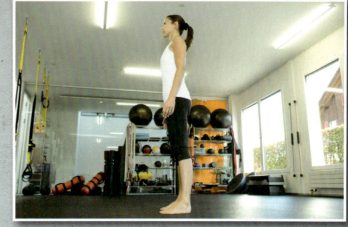

Motion: Start by bending your knees and at the same time, moving your buttocks backwards as if you wanted to sit down in a chair. Keep your torso upright and chest out. While lowering down, raise your arms up to help you balance. Bring your buttocks down to knee level or lower, keeping your upper body as upright as possible.

Easier alternative: Hold on to something while doing this exercise and don't go down as low.

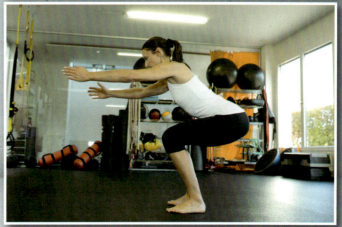

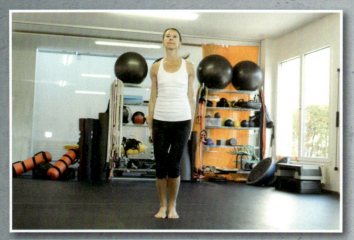

JUMPING JACK

Starting position: Stand up straight and upright. Feet close together, arms at your side.

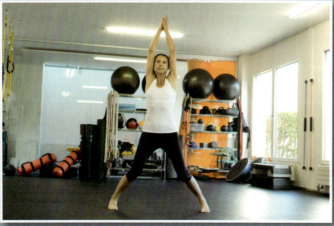

Motion: Jump up and bring your legs out to the side. At the same time, raise your arms over your head and clap your hands. Jump back to the starting position. Repeat in a controlled tempo.

20-MINUTE HIGH INTENSIVE INTERVAL TRAINING (HIIT)
Do as many rounds as you can for 20 minutes

1ST ROUND
200m sprint
5 handstand push-ups
5 pull-ups
10 squats
(no rest)

ROUND 2
100m sprint
10 handstand push-ups
10 pull-ups
20 squats
(no rest)

ROUND 3
200m sprint
15 handstand push-ups
15 pull-ups
30 squats
(no rest)

ROUND 4
100m sprint
20 handstand push-ups
20 pull-ups
40 squats
(no rest)

ROUND 5
200m sprint
25 handstand push-ups
25 pull-ups
50 squats
(no rest)

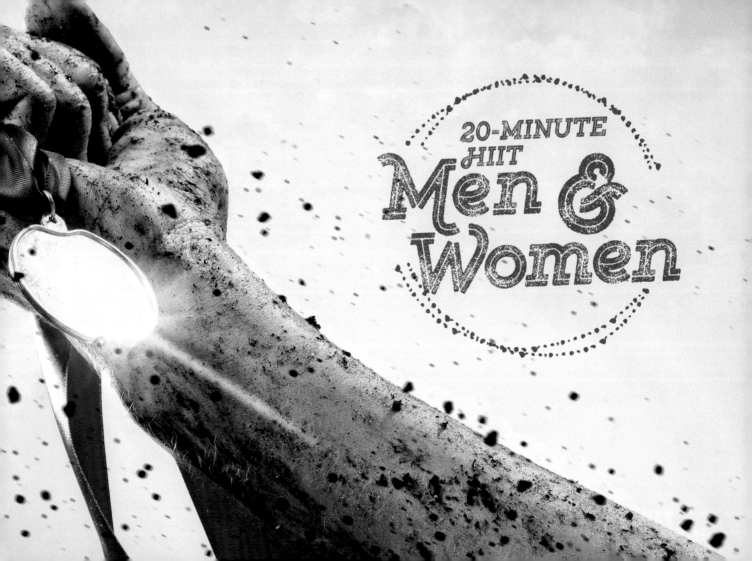

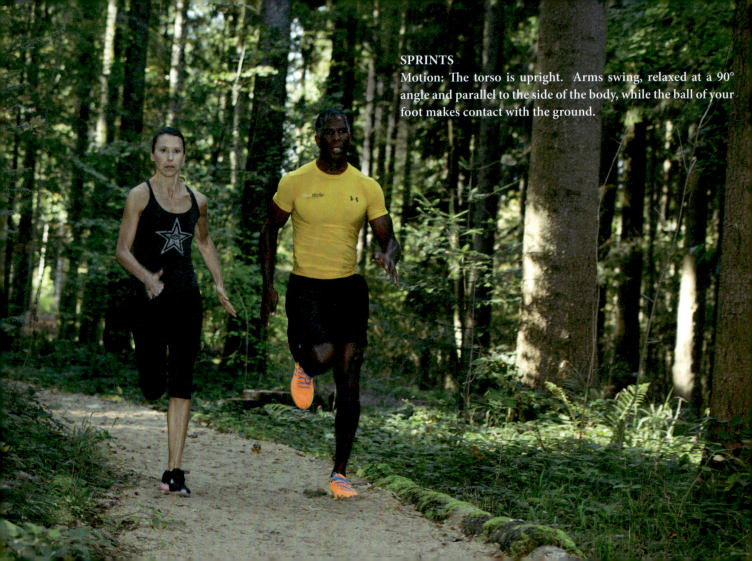

SPRINTS
Motion: The torso is upright. Arms swing, relaxed at a 90° angle and parallel to the side of the body, while the ball of your foot makes contact with the ground.

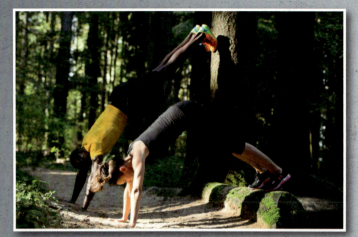

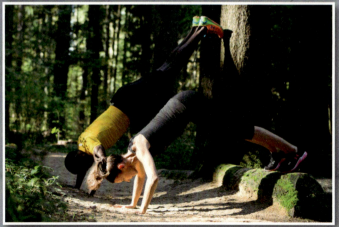

HANDSTAND PUSH-UP

Beginner starting position: Place your feet on an elevated non-slip surface. From here, go into the push-up position. Hands are shoulder-width apart under your chest. Push your buttocks up as high as you can. Knees are fully extended and back is straight.

Advanced starting position: Go into the push up position and put your feet up on a wall. Now walk up the wall with your feet, paying attention to keep your abdomen muscles tensed.

Motion: Bend your arms slowly so that your head moves toward the floor. Focus on body tension. From this position, push yourself back up to the starting position with your arms.

PULL-UPS HORIZONTAL
(see description on page 192)

PULL-UPS VERTICAL
Starting position, the easier alternative (Romy, *left*): Hands shoulder-width apart, grip the bar with an underhand grip.

Starting position, the advanced alternative (Dave, *right*): Hands shoulder-width apart, grip the bar with an overhand grip.

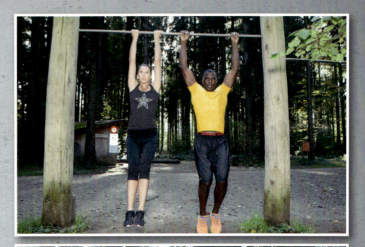

How to do a pull-up correctly: Beginning with arms stretched, pull yourself up until your chin is above the bar. Slowly return to starting position (arms stretched).

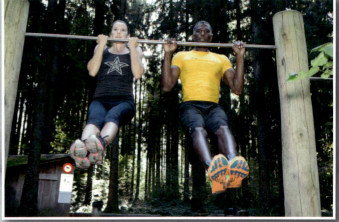

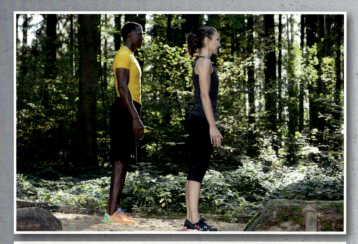

SQUAT

Starting Position: Stand straight with your feet parallel and hip-width apart.

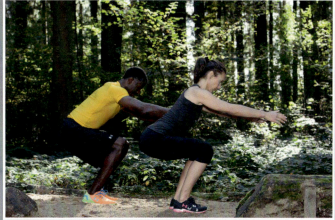

Motion: Start by bending your knees while at the same time moving your buttocks backwards, as if you wanted to sit down in a chair. Keep your torso upright and chest out. While lowering down, bring your arms up to help you balance. Bring your buttocks down to knee level or lower, keeping your torso as upright as possible.

Beginners may hold on to something for support.

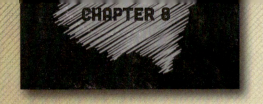

Sources
AND INFORMATION

FRUIT BELLY

PURE FOOD PRODUCTS

STORE (ONLINE)	PRODUCTS
Swanson Vitamins http://www.swansonvitamins.com/	Coconut products, cacao products, nut butter, ghee
EVitamins http://www.evitamins.com/	Cacao, nut butters, coconut oil
Lucky Vitamin http://www.luckyvitamin.com/	Coconut products, cacao products, nuts, gelatin, ghee
iHerb http://www.iherb.com/	Coconut products, cacao, herbs, supplements, everything paleo
Coconut Secret https://www.coconutsecret.com/products2.html	Coconut products like coconut vinegar, crystals, flour, oil, etc.
Vitamin Shoppe http://www.vitaminshoppe.com/	Supplements, superfoods, everything paleo
VitaCost www.vitacost.com	Nut butter, ghee, raw honey, chia, superfoods, supplements, everything and anything paleo

You can find organic meat and fish, as well as vegetables in an organic health food store or in larger grocery stores. Health food stores such as Whole Foods, Trader Joe's, and Sprouts, as well as local co-ops, farmer's markets, and CSAs offer a wide selection of good quality organic products.

You can find coconut products in health food stores or in the previously mentioned online shops. In the US, online retailers that specialize in healthy products, such as iHerb, Vitacost, Swanson Vitamins, and the Vitamin Shoppe all sell organic, high quality coconut-based products. Thrive Market, a membership based program, is a great option for those looking to keep their budget low, as the service combines top quality organic products at more affordable prices.

Key words that may indicate good quality:
- Organic
- Raw
- Extra virgin

A weekly trip to the farmers market or buying directly from a local farmer will make shopping a fun experience.

PURE FOOD BASIC INFORMATION

VCO

Virgin Coconut Oil is cold-pressed coconut oil. It has a high content of short chain fatty acids and does not require bile or digestive enzymes to be digested. This relieves the digestion considerably. High quality coconut oil also has a high content of lauric acid, which is found naturally in breast milk. Coconut oil is practically free of omega-6 fatty acids and is also cholesterol free. Avoid hydrogenated coconut oil products that are available in many discount grocery stores, often found next to the lard and other cheap cooking oils and shortenings. Coconut oil can be heated to very high temperatures, which makes it perfect for frying. It becomes solid if it is stored at temperatures below 77° F, and liquid at temperatures over 77° F.

EXTRA VIRGIN OLIVE OIL

Cold pressed olive oil has been used since ancient times due to its health-promoting properties. The content of polyunsaturated fatty acids is very high. Oleic acid is also dominant in olive oil. High quality products are labeled extra virgin, cold pressed, or first cold pressed. There has been a lot of controversy on the quality of olive oil. Olive oil should never be heated to high temperatures since the fatty acids become saturated and harmful to your health. It's best used cold…dribbled on your food or used in salad dressings. Gently heating it at low temperatures is fine.

INSTANT GELATIN

Gelatin is pure protein obtained from collagen-containing raw materials such as bone, cartilage, connective tissue, and minerals. Gelatin is available in powder form or is pressed into thin transparent sheets (sheet or leaf gelatin). It contains 18 different amino acids, including all essential amino acids with the exception of tryptophan.

We are familiar with using gelatin in the kitchen as a thickening agent. It's used in desserts such as Jell-O and panna cotta, and is also used when making savory dishes such as aspic. We are less familiar with using gelatin as a supplement, often referred to as instant gelatin.

Instant gelatin has no taste, is water-soluble in cold water, and will not thicken into a gel-like substance. It supplies the body with essential nutrients for the ongoing regeneration of the cartilage in our joints, hair, skin, connective tissue, and nails. About 40 percent of total protein in the human body consists of collagen, which is mainly found in the skin and connective tissue.

You can make gelatin yourself at home by brewing your own bone broth—by cooking bones for several hours. While the broth is cooking, you won't see the gelatin. Once you allow the broth to cool, the protein will gel, turning the liquid broth into a gelatinous mass.

HIGH QUALITY CACAO PRODUCTS *(chocolate, cocoa powder, and cocoa nibs containing more than 80 percent cacao)*

In ancient Latin America, cocoa was regarded as extremely valuable. Cocoa beans were used as currency in the Mayan civilization. And the Aztecs kept the brown beans as an offering to the feathered serpent god called Quetzalcoatl. As good and valuable as cocoa may be, we must use it in moderation. High quality cocoa powder is not chocolate powder. High quality cocoa powder or cocoa nibs (chopped cocoa beans) taste more bitter, astringent, and are not sweet. High quality cocoa contains a large amount of antioxidants.

COCONUT FLOUR

Coconut flour is made of the dried meat of coconuts. It is gluten free, rich in fiber, and low in carbohydrates. Coconut flour can be used as a flour substitute when baking, however it doesn't have the same baking properties as conventional flour, necessitating more liquid when used for baking.

TAMARI

Tamari is the traditional gluten free soy sauce. In industrially produced soy sauce, wheat is used for the brewing process. Tamari is made purely of fermented soybeans and salt, with no added wheat.

GHEE

Ghee is a type of clarified butter, also called butter fat. Butter is carefully heated and left to simmer for about 30 minutes, without allowing it to brown. The proteins in the butter become curdled, forming a white foam on the top that eventually sinks to the bottom of the pan when the water evaporates. The butter becomes clarified by skimming the foam off while cooking and/or filtering it after cooking. Lactose and casein (milk protein) are eliminated in this process. Ghee contains the high quality short fatty acids of milk and is, along with coconut oil, one of the easiest to digest fats. In Indian cuisine, ghee is considered liquid gold due to its health benefits.

SWEET POTATOES

Botanically speaking, sweet potatoes are not actually a potato; they can be eaten raw. In China, Japan, USA, and South America, they are a staple food. In Europe, sweet potatoes have a shadowy existence. You can use sweet potatoes as you would potatoes, however they have quite different nutritional factors. Depending on the variety, sweet potatoes contain substantial amounts of beta-carotene, vitamin A, B6, C, thiamine, and potassium.

RAW DAIRY PRODUCTS

Depending on where you live, you may be able to buy raw milk or raw milk products, such as cheese and butter. Raw milk is not pasteurized or otherwise heated, and is not homogenized. By heating milk, essential vitamins and enzymes are lost, not to mention the breaking down of the fat molecules, making it difficult for the body to digest. If you are lactose intolerant, it's better to avoid raw milk and its products. Fresh, unripened cheese (mozzarella, ricotta, cream cheese) and naturally aged cheese (parmesan, cheddar) are usually well tolerated. Raw milk products are easy to digest and are an excellent source for protein, vitamins, calcium, and fat.

MACADAMIA NUTS

Macadamia nuts, besides coconuts, contain the lowest amount of omega-6 fatty acids. And macadamia nuts have by far the highest fat content of all nuts. Real Pure Food!

PROTEIN POWDER

Protein powder keeps popping up in recipes (especially in smoothie recipes). You might have an image in your head when you think of protein powder—of a bodybuilding store, the shelves loaded with big tubs of all different kinds of protein powder. Don't worry, protein powder does not equal bodybuilding or doping. Depending on the manufacturer, it's a great, simple, and safe way to get high quality protein.

But not all protein powders are the same! There are many different kinds of protein powders out there: whey-based, casein-based, and vegan protein powders—rice, pea and hemp-based.

You're probably asking yourself, which one you should choose? I advise you to take whey isolate!

Whey is a protein with high biological value, is well absorbed by the body, and easily digested. Casein (milk protein), and egg protein as well, could cause digestive problems. Soy protein is mostly made of genetically manipulated soybeans and beef protein may not come from happy/healthy organically reared cows. You should also pay attention to the lactose content of the various protein powders. It's best to choose a lactose-free product (casein or whey concentrate also contains a lot of lactose). We'll go into more detail on this.

To make it even more complicated, there are many different methods in which whey is produced. The best quality whey is made by cross-flow microfiltration (CMF). We don't recommend ion-exchange whey.

The higher the quality of the whey, the less amounts of residual lactose it will contain. Really high quality whey will be practically lactose-free.

BRAND	PRODUCT	AVAILABLE AT:
Optimum Nutrition	Gold Standard 100% Whey	www.luckyvitamin.com, www.iherb.com
NOW Foods	Whey Protein	www.swansonvitamins.com, www.vitaminshoppe.com
Biochem	Natural Whey Protein Isolate	www.thrivemarket.com, www.vitacost.com

FRUCTOSE AND FODMAP FOOD LIST

0 allowed   **1** less than 100 grams (3.5 oz) allowed   **2** avoid

Food	Fructose (per 100 grams)	FODMAP
Apple	5.74	2
Apricot	0.09	2
Artichoke	1.73	2
Asparagus	0.99	2
Asparagus, canned	0.57	2
Avocado	0.20	1
Banana	3.40	0
Beets	0.50	2
Belgian endive	0.68	0
Blackberries	3.11	2
Blueberries	3.35	1
Broccoli	1.04	1
Broccoli, cooked	0.80	1
Brussels sprouts	0.79	1
Brussels sprouts, cooked	0.54	1
Cabbage, Chinese	0.51	0
Cabbage, green	0.92	0
Cabbage, savoy	0.90	0
Cabbage, white	1.76	0
Carrots	1.31	1
Carrots, cooked	0.94	1
Cauliflower	0.86	2
Cauliflower, cooked	0.76	2
Celeriac	0.10	1
Chard	0.270	0
Cherries	6.1	2
Cranberries	2.93	1
Cucumber	0.86	0
Currants, black	3.07	1
Currants, red	2.49	1
Currants, white	3.00	1
Dandelion leaves	0.555	0
Eggplant	1.03	0
Endive	0.60	0
Fennel	1.06	1
Figs	23.5	2
Gooseberries	3.33	2
Grapefruit	2.10	2
Grapes	7.44	0
Honey	40.0	2

FRUIT BELLY

	Fructose (per 100 grams)	FODMAP
Honeydew melon	1.30	0
Kiwi	4.6	0
Kohlrabi	1.23	1
Leek	1.23	2
Lemon	1.35	0
Lemon juice	1.03	0
Lettuce	0.53	0
Lime	0.80	0
Litchi	3.20	2
Mango	2.60	2
Mushrooms	0.21	2
Mushrooms, chanterelle	0.07	1
Mushrooms, portobello	0.26	2
Okra	0.80	0
Onion	1.34	2
Orange	2.58	0
Papaya	0.33	0
Parsley, leaf	0.32	0
Parsley, root	0.66	0
Parsnip	0.26	0
Passion fruit	3.96	0
Peach	1.23	2

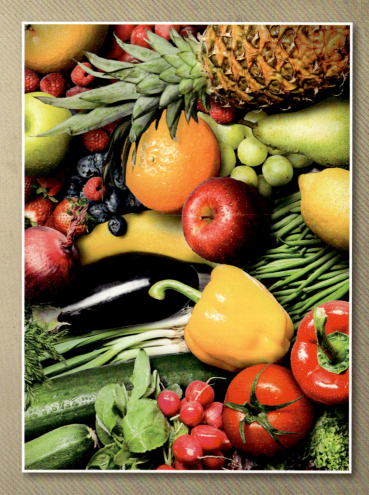

	Fructose (per 100 grams)	FODMAP
Pear	6.7	2
Persimmon	5.56	2
Pineapple	2.44	0
Plum	2.01	2
Potato	0.17	0
Prickly pear	0.60	0
Pumpkin	1.32	1
Radish, daikon	0.60	1
Radishes	0.72	1
Raspberries	2.05	1
Rhubarb	0.39	0
Sauerkraut	0.20	2
Sauerkraut, drained	0.21	2
Spinach	0.12	0
Strawberries	2.30	0
Sweet potatoes	0.66	2
Tangerine	1.30	0
Tomato	1.36	0
Tomato, canned	1.25	0
Watermelon	3.92	2
Zucchini	1.02	1

RAW MILK PRODUCTS CONTAINING LACTOSE

	Lactose (per 100 grams)	FODMAP
Milk (cow's, sheep, goat's)	4.9	0
Cream	3.5	1
Butter	Traces	0
Camembert cheese	None	0
Brie	None	0
Semi-hard cheese		
Cheddar	None	0
Hard and extra hard cheese		
Parmesan	None	0
Pecorino	None	0

GRAINS AND POSSIBLE USES

	Gluten	FODMAP
Wheat (Pasta, bread, baked goods)	Yes	2
Durum wheat (Pasta, couscous)	Yes	2
Rye (Bread, baked goods)	Yes	2
Barley, green spelt	Yes	2
Kamut, emmer wheat	Yes	2
Spelt (Bread, pasta, baked goods)	Yes	0
Oats	Traces	0
Rice (Pure, crackers, noodles)	No	0
Buckwheat (Flour, pure)	No	0
Quinoa (Pure, pasta)	No	0
Amaranth (Pure, pops)	No	0
Potatoes	No	0
Sweet potatoes	No	2
Maize (Polenta)	No	0
Chestnuts	No	0
Teff (lovegrass)	No	0
Millet	No	0

NUTS/SEEDS

	FODMAP
Almonds	2
Cashews	2
Hazelnuts	2
Macadamia nuts	0
Pecans	0
Pine nuts	0
Pistachios	2
Chia seeds	0
Pumpkin seeds	0
Sesame seeds	0
Sunflower seeds	0
Walnuts	0
Tempeh	0

PAY ATTENTION TO: MUSTARD, BOUILLON POWDERS, SAUCE THICKENERS, DRIED FIGS, SALAMI, VEGETARIAN MEAT-SUBSTITUTES

Appendix

QUICK FIX SHOPPING LIST

FOR THE PANTRY:
Instant gelatin, olive oil, salt, pepper, butter
Optional: nutmeg, turmeric, cinnamon, cardamom, coconut oil, sesame seeds

WHAT TO BUY (FOR ONE PERSON):
- 2 cups coconut milk
- Fresh ginger
- 2 lemon grass stalks
- Chili
- Thai basil
- 1 bunch chives
- 1 bunch parsley
- 1 avocado
- At least 1 lb beets, steamed
- 2 packages steamed carrots plus 1 lb fresh carrots or 1 lb fresh carrots
- 2 lb sweet potatoes
- 1 lb potatoes
- 1 lb fresh spinach
- ¼ lb eggplant
- ¼ lb zucchini
- ¼ lb pumpkin
- ¼ lb celeriac
- ½ lb canned tomatoes
- ¾ lb chicken breast (without skin)
- ¼ lb thinly sliced cutlets
- ¼ lb ground beef (not lean)
- ¼ lb diced veal
- ¼ lb salmon filet
- ¼ lb canned tuna fish (in salt water)

EQUIPMENT SUPPLIERS

NAME	INTERNET ADDRESS OF MANUFACTURER
Nike+ Fuelband	http://www.nike.com/us/en_us/c/nikeplus-fuel
Fitbit One	http://www.fitbit.com/one
Jawbone UP MOVE	https://jawbone.com/

Acknowledgments

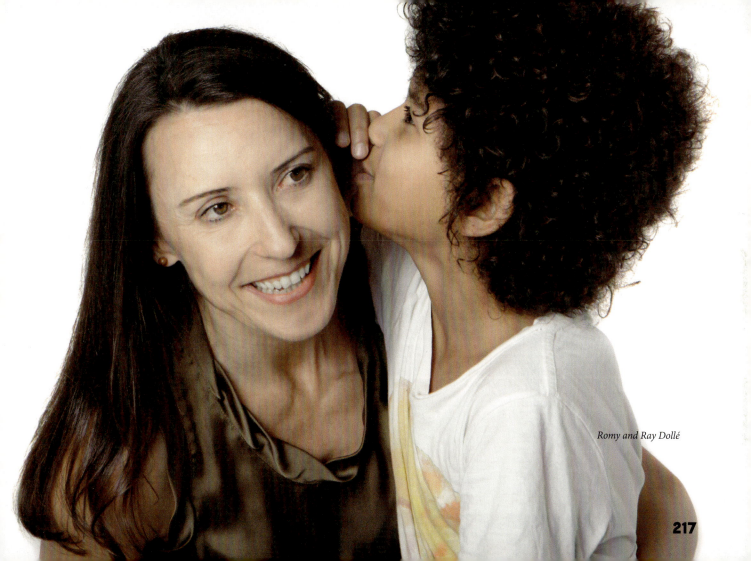

Romy and Ray Dollé

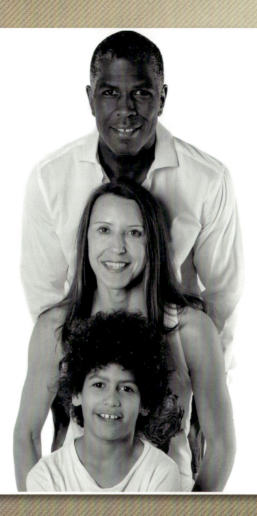

Dave, Romy, and Ray Dollé

I thank my husband Dave and my son Ray for their support. They have been my most critical recipe testers. Dave and I have big discussions about lifestyle issues. We do the research together and have evolved both individually and in our life philosophy together. I appreciate this very much and am grateful that we can enjoy this experience and knowledge together. Ray is my sunshine and makes me smile many times a day. We have daily discussions on where the boundaries are. We may have stubborn arguments, but we make up with warm hugs.

In order to take my ideas for this book and turn them into a finished product, I received generous support from four bright minds. We were a motivated team made up of very different characters. It was lots of fun. I'd like to thank:

Sibylla—for her in-depth research, her eloquent writing style, and tireless efforts. She is well on her way to becoming a successful journalist/author herself.

Nadine E.—for her great knowledge on diet and nutrition. I can ask her anything and will always get an immediate answer. She's the one who asked critical questions about many of the topics in this book. This has not always been fun, but it definitely improved this book and always pushed me to the limits. Nadine took over the tasks that required perfection and precision. The creative staff was grateful for this.

Nadine G.—for her most incredible joy and enthusiasm. She invested her heart and soul into the topics of belly shapes, fitness, and stress. We all benefited from her cheerful mood and incorporated it into this book.

Torsten—for his medical and scientific explanations. He was able to make the difficult subjects more understandable for all of us. Torsten also reviewed the entire manuscript for accuracy.

I owe a huge thank you to my esteemed German publisher, Sabine Schmieder, for her trust in me and my ideas. Our work together was, from the beginning, very professional and constructive.

Many thanks to Fabian Seiler (www.fabian-seiler.ch), who shared his experiences with us and allowed us to have a deeper look inside.

In the final phase of the book, when I somehow lost focus and ambition (according to the Pareto-Principle, 80 percent is more than enough) Gabrielle came into my life. She taught me to accept my fatigue, my aversion to work on the manuscript, my lack of patience, and my fear of not being able to deliver a perfect book—to just accept it all and let it go. I experienced intense moments in her neurofeedback-training and was able to free myself, accept, and move forward in a brilliant final sprint. For this, I would like to thank Gabrielle.

I am also greatly appreciative of the interest expressed by Mark Sisson and Brad Kearns, my friends at Primal Blueprint Publishing, for translating my original work, *Früchtewampe*, for the US market. After being enthusiastic followers of the Primal Blueprint for many years, Dave and I had the pleasure of meeting Mark and Brad in person at the PrimalCon event in Tulum, Mexico, in March of 2014, then again in Los Angeles in 2015 when the English edition approached publication.

Thanks also to you, dear reader. I am happy to answer any questions you may have. My contact details may be found on my website: www.romydolle.com

Epilogue

You've made it this far. You've read the whole book, possibly tried some things out. Or maybe you've skipped from the introduction to the last word, glancing at a few of the photos. There is no general rule on how to read this book or how to live your life. What is important is that you find a way to make yourself happy and content. Don't forget, health is the foundation of a happy life. If you are aware of this, it will be easier to make many decisions.

I have learned a lot since I started to think about this book and its contents. I have grown and reached a new level—a process that never seems to end. I read many books and blog articles about health, fitness, diet, fasting, and meditation.

In the past few years, I decided to undertake meditating. I tried all different types of meditation, but I was never able to find peace with my inner self and slide into the depths of relaxation. I found over the years that I am better able to relax while walking. With the steady steps, the relaxation of my hips spreads to my pelvis, abdomen, chest, shoulders, and all the way up to my head. After about 20 minutes, I'm in the flow and I really enjoy it. It may sound funny, but this is exactly how I feel. I'm simply happy that I can be alone with myself and I can feel myself. I'm aware of the air and the temperature on my skin and I feel the ground under my feet. At that moment, everything is okay. I am in the here and now.

Shortly before I started with the manuscript for this book, I was able to take a break from work. I suddenly had so much more time to write. I was able to plan my days the way I wanted to. This was nice, but on the other hand, I wasn't used to it. I didn't have structured days anymore. Everything was free-flowing and flexible. I enjoyed this for a few weeks, but the manuscript somehow lost its place on my schedule. I had so many other interests and exciting people with whom I'd rather spend my time.

So I gave my days new structure. I had a morning ritual: get up early, short intense workout, read for 20 minutes, meditate for seven minutes, write in my appreciation journal, make a "to do list" for the day. This took about an hour and was a good foundation for the rest of the day. One hour for me alone—doing something for my body, mind, and soul.

I started a new experiment with meditating. I would set a small goal and would begin with meditating for one minute. It took a few days until I was able to sit or lie on the floor and not let the thoughts come into my head. Slowly, I was able to increase my time up to seven minutes. It's been a few weeks already since I've reached 7 minutes, and it'll take me a bit longer before I can meditate longer. To be completely relaxed for just two or five minutes gives me so much more room in my head. I'm able to clear and rearrange my mind.

By establishing my morning routine, I got in the habit of meditating in the mornings. Sometimes during the day, I long for the feeling I get while meditating—that clear and relaxed feeling in my head. And just the thought of this will relax me. I'm grateful, even after so many unsuccessful attempts, to have managed to learn how to meditate.

Every morning my appreciation journal shows me the positive aspects of my life and this feeling of gratitude remains with me all day. I write nearly everyday in my journal—I'm grateful that I am healthy, that I slept well, and that my husband and son are both healthy. And then many other things will come to mind, people and experiences that I am grateful for.

This may sound completely mundane; it is a very simple exercise. However, the effect it has on my confidence and my satisfaction is extremely impressive. Problems and concerns are put into perspective, not ignored. The good things in life are valued. Starting your day with the positive aspects of your life will help you be more relaxed throughout the day.

In a relaxed state, I'm able to make better decisions, I'm less stressed, and I'm able to use my energy more meaningfully.

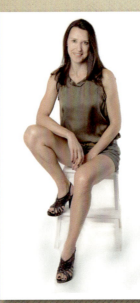

"YES, I'M HAPPY. NO, I'M NOT PERFECT."

Romy

Contributors

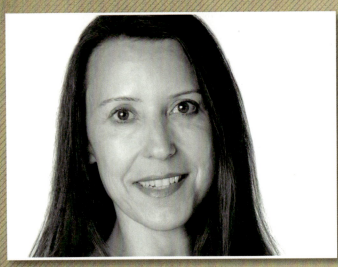
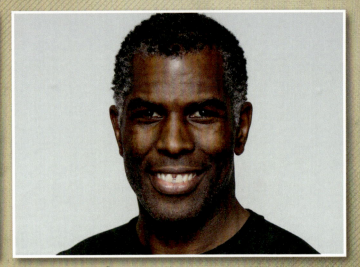

ROMY DOLLÉ

Married to Dave Dollé and mother of Ray (b.2005). Family woman and entrepreneur, Swiss-certified banking specialist/MBA, and author.

Romy is curious and adventurous. She's willing to take risks while always keeping an eye on her family's financial security. She loves to discover new places, have new experiences, to observe and meet new people—while maintaining and appreciating existing friendships, in the knowledge that love and freedom can perfectly coexist.

DAVE DOLLÉ

Married to Romy Dollé and father of Ray, Dave is a former top-ranking athlete (100 and 200 meters sprint). Today, he is a Swiss-known fitness expert, trainer, entrepreneur, and frequent spokesperson/international keynote speaker and fitness presenter.

Optimally combining fun and exercise, Dave enjoys going snowboarding with his family, skiing in the Alps, making his city's skatepark "unsafe" by trying teenage tricks as an older guy, and hitting the golf ball 340 yards!

Dave is always focused on the "why". He optimizes efficiency when organizing his daily agenda and has a strong ability to maintain alertness while still remaining relaxed.

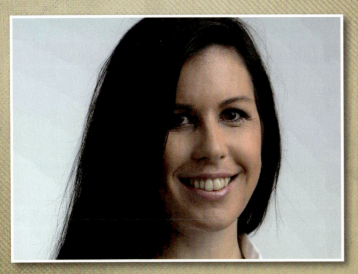 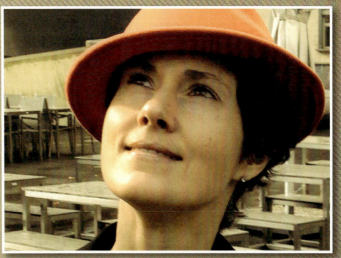

SIBYLLA ROTZLER

Sibylla studies journalism and corporate publishing at the School of Applied Linquistics (SAL) in Zürich and works at SIX Group for Corporate Communications, when not writing blog posts for Dave Dollé and and leading the editorial department. After graduating from the Higher School of Tourism (HFT) in Luzern, she explored the world as a flight attendant and got to experience the cultures and countries of the world. Knowledge of the power of thought drives her to learn more about people and their behavior. Sport and diet keep her in balance, so that she has power and energy for everyday life. With power yoga, she is able to find not only relaxation, but also the necessary amount of fitness.

NADINE ESPOSITO

A fascination for questions concerning diet and sport brought Nadine Esposito and Romy together. Years of struggling with food intolerances led her to come to terms with food and its composition, and her compulsion is now her passion. Nadine would like to help spread the message that nutrition does not have to be a struggle, but a central aspect of life and the foundation for good health. Food should give you energy, sensuality, and joy.

"It's been a pleasure to be able to support Romy with her books **Good Fat, Bad Fat** and **Fruit Belly**." N.E.

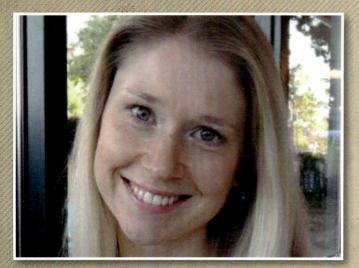

NADINE GERETZKY

(Junior personal trainer at www.davedolle.com)

A passion for fitness led Nadine to Dave Dollé and Pure Training, where she realized her dream of becoming a personal trainer. Originally educated in social work (BA) with an emphasis on disease prevention and promotion of health, she completed additional training to become a specialist in corporate health management. Her work reflects her deep interest in the extremely complex interaction between the body, mind, and soul. Nadine has conducted various personal experiments with different types of diets to define the best personal health regimen possible. She's found that delicious, healthy/natural food, intense strength and fitness training, and restorative relaxation best allow her to be a happy and balanced person.

Nadine loves to inspire people with her enthusiasm for a healthy lifestyle, to make them laugh and give them strength to find their own way to achieve their individual goals.

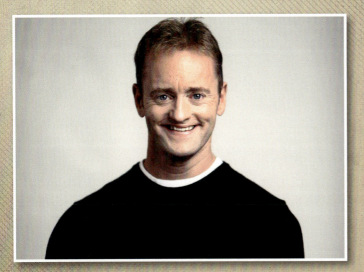

DR. TORSTEN ALBERS, M.D.

Albers concept, Zürich/Schlieren, www.albers-concepts.com

As a former athlete with a PhD in sports dietetics, experience working with amateur and professional athletes in the areas of training and diet, Dr. Torsten Albers provides expertise on nutrition, medicine, and training to his customers and patients.

His clientele spans athletes in the martial arts, triathletes, ice hockey players, performers, fitness enthusiasts, and those trying to lose weight to people with medical problems. He also brings comprehensive health coaching to entrepreneurs and executives who would like to restore or improve their physical and mental fitness and performance.

The original edition of *Früchtewampe*, published in German, has many footnotes and references not included in this version. If you want to review any source material for validation, you can visit the author's website: http://romydolle.com/cms/. It will be in German, but Google will translate for you.

Additional Photography and Illustration Credits:

Background of pages 8 – 121: © kantver - Fotolia.com
Background of pages 122 – 125, S. 204-228: creativemarket.com
Background of pages 126 – 179: © Alx - Fotolia.com
Background of pages 180 – 203: © kantver - Fotolia.com
Pages 10, 56, 60, 73, 211: © lassedesignen - Fotolia.com
Pages 12, 15, 34, 55, 117, 118: © olly - Fotolia.com
Pages 13/14: © SeDmi - shutterstock.com
Page 16: © Jenny Sturm - Fotolia.com
Page 17: © librakv - Shutterstock.com
Page 29: creativemarket.com
Page 32: © babimu - Fotolia.com
Page 35: © Stockphoto4u - iStockphoto.com
Page 36 Illustration: Anneke Reiß-Maaoui, Bremen
Page 37: © Valentina R. - Fotolia.com
Page 39: © Maksim Smeljov - Fotolia.com
Page 42: © LoloStock - Fotolia.com
Page 46: © MedinaMedina - iStockphoto.com
Page 47: © HandmadePictures - Fotolia.com
Page 52: © fox17 - Fotolia.com
Page 54: © Michael Kempf - Fotolia.com
Page 55: © Africa Studio - Fotolia.com
Page 57: © Thomas Neumahr - Fotolia.com
Page 58: © Okea - Fotolia.com
Page 62: © AlexPro9500 - iStockphoto.com
Page 67: © bilderzwerg - Fotolia.com
Page 69: © ra2studio - Fotolia.com
Page 71: © Kemalbas - iStockphoto.com

Page 72: © Mayer George - shutterstock.com
Page 74: © FotoKachna - Fotolia.com
Page 76: © Mariday - Fotolia.com
Page 79: Photodisc
Page 83: © Sergey Nivens - Fotolia.com
Page 84: © 2007 Ron Chapple Stock - Fotolia.com
Page 88: © Kurhan - Fotolia.com
Page 90: © Sergejs Rahunoks @ YekoPhotoStudio - Fotolia.com
Page 94: © Diana Taliun - iStockphoto.com
Page 95: © underdogstudios - Fotolia.com
Page 97: © drubig-photo - Fotolia.com
Page 101: © kesipun - shutterstock.com
Page 104: © 4774344sean - iStockphoto.com
Page 105: © Martin Benik - Fotolia.com
Page 106: © contrastwerkstatt - Fotolia.com
Page 107: © Nikita Buida - Fotolia.com
Page 107: © peterjunaidy - Fotolia.com
Page 108 Illustration: Anneke Reiß-Maaoui, Bremen
Page 110: © Ovidiu Iordachi - Fotolia.com
Page 114: © Monkey Business - Fotolia.com
Page 120: © Maygutyak - Fotolia.com
Page 121: © Beba73 - iStockphoto.com
Page 130: © Warren Goldswain - Fotolia.com
Page 144: © EcoPim-studio - Fotolia.com
Page 190: © Kuzma - shutterstock.com
Page 194: © Mariday - Fotolia.com
Pages 198/199: © Sergey Nivens - Fotolia.com

OTHER BOOKS BY PRIMAL BLUEPRINT PUBLISHING

MARK SISSON

The Primal Connection: Follow your genetic blueprint to health and happiness

The Primal Blueprint: Reprogram your genes for effortless weight loss, vibrant health, and boundless energy

The Primal Blueprint 21-Day Total Body Transformation: A step-by-step diet and lifestyle makeover to become a fat-burning machine!

The Primal Blueprint 90-Day Journal: A Personal Experiment (n=1)

COOKBOOKS BY MARK SISSON AND JENNIFER MEIER

The Primal Blueprint Cookbook: Primal, low carb, paleo, grain-free, dairy-free and gluten-free meals

The Primal Blueprint Quick and Easy Meals: Delicous, Primal-approved meals you can make in under 30 minutes

The Primal Blueprint Healthy Sauces, Dressings, and Toppings: Plus rubs, dips, marinades and other easy ways to transform basic natural foods into Primal masterpieces

OTHER AUTHORS

Hidden Plague: *A field guide for surviving and overcoming hidradenitis suppurativa,* by Tara Grant

Rich Food, Poor Food: *The Ultimate Grocery Purchasing System (GPS),* by Mira Calton, CN, and Jayson Calton, Ph.D.

Death by Food Pyramid: *How shoddy science, sketchy politics and shady special interests ruined your health,* by Denise Minger

The South Asian Health Solution: *A culturally tailored guide to lose fat, increase energy, avoid disease,* by Ronesh Sinha, MD

Paleo Girl: *A straight talk guide to navigating the challenges of adolescence with a sensible, stress-balanced, Primal approach,* by Leslie Klenke

Lil' Grok Meets the Korgs: *A prehistoric boy shows a high tech modern family how to live Primally,* by Janée Meadows

COOKBOOKS

The Paleo Primer: *A jump-start guide to losing body fat and living Primally,* by Keris Marsden and Matt Whitmore

Primal Cravings: *Your favorite foods made paleo,* by Brandon and Megan Keatley